CHAKRA HEALING FOR BEGINNERS

How to Heal and Balance Your Chakras Through Meditation

Yoga, Gemstones and Crystals. Positive Energy, Awareness therapy

Buddhism Principles, and Psychic Development

© Spiritual Awakening Academy

Text Copyright © Spiritual Awakening Academy

All rights reserved. No part of this guide may be reproduced in any form without permission in writing from the publisher except in the case of brief quotations embodied in critical articles or reviews.

Legal & Disclaimer

The information contained in this book and its contents is not designed to replace or take the place of any form of medical or professional advice; and is not meant to replace the need for independent medical, financial, legal or other professional advice or services, as may be required. The content and information in this book has been provided for educational and entertainment purposes only.

The content and information contained in this book has been compiled from sources deemed reliable, and it is accurate to the best of the Author's knowledge, information and belief. However, the Author cannot guarantee its accuracy and validity and cannot be held liable for any errors and/or omissions. Further, changes are periodically made to this book as and when needed. Where appropriate and/or necessary, you must consult a professional (including but not limited to your doctor, attorney, financial advisor or such other professional advisor) before using any of the suggested remedies, techniques, or information in this book.

Upon using the contents and information contained in this book, you agree to hold harmless the Author from and against any damages, costs, and expenses, including any legal fees potentially resulting from the application of any of the information provided by this book. This disclaimer applies to any loss, damages or injury caused by the use and application, whether directly or indirectly, of any advice or information presented, whether for breach of contract, tort, negligence, personal injury, criminal intent, or under any other cause of action.

You agree to accept all risks of using the information presented inside this book.

You agree that by continuing to read this book, where appropriate and/or necessary, you shall consult a professional (including but not limited to your doctor, attorney, or financial advisor or such other advisor as needed) before using any of the suggested remedies, techniques, or information in this book.

Table of Contents

INTRODUCTION — 5

CHAPTER 1: A BRIEF HISTORY ON CHAKRAS — 8

CHAPTER 2: BASIC CHAKRA TRUTHS — 12

CHAPTER 3: GUIDED CHAKRA MEDITATION FOR BEGINNERS — 23

- *Common mistakes*
- *1. Get started with a daily meditation routine.*
- *2. Fall asleep*
- *3. Finding it difficult to hold the focus*
- *4. Not preparing your meditation environment:*
- *5. Force yourself*
- *6. Not setting a daily time for meditation:*
- *7. Set too high expectations for yourself*

CHAPTER 4: THE BENEFIT OF THE DIFFERENT CHAKRAS — 39

CHAPTER 5: CRYSTAL HEALING FOR CHAKRAS — 46

- MEDITATION FOR THE SACRAL CHAKRA
- MEDITATION FOR THE SOLAR PLEXUS CHAKRA
- MEDITATION FOR THE HEART CHAKRA
- MEDITATION FOR THE THROAT CHAKRA
- MEDITATION FOR THE THIRD EYE CHAKRA

CHAPTER 6: CHAKRAS ENERGY SYSTEM- LIVING WITH YOUR OWN ENERGY — 118

CHAPTER 7: SOME YOGA EXERCISES — 123

CHAPTER 8: THE HINDU AND THE BUDDHIST TANTRAS — 133

CHAPTER 9: KEEPING BALANCE: BREATHING PRACTICES CONCLUSION — 153

Introduction

Welcome to **Chakras for Beginners:** A Complete Guide to Balance Chakras and Healing Yourself with Crystals and Meditation for Health and Positive Energy!

How much do you already know about your chakras? If you are reading this book, then you probably have a lot of questions that need answering and you are in luck because this guide is here to show you the way. There are so many wonderful ways that you can explore not just your physical health, but your emotional and mental health as well.

The history of the chakras is ancient and comes from another culture that accurately described the essence of our "subtle bodies". If you practice yoga, you might know a thing or two about these concepts because the same culture that invented yoga practices, also wrote about our chakras and how they work. In this book, you will learn more about the history of how chakras came to be known, and how we are only just learning about the science behind them in our western culture.

You will learn about the individual chakras that make up the main chakra system, as well as the additional chakras that can exist at other points in your body. It is important that as you learn more about each of these "energy centers" that you know how they can impact your overall health. This guide will give you explanations for how your chakras can become imbalanced or blocked and why that can cause physical, emotional, and mental side effects.

You want to know how to heal those blocks and imbalances and this book is the perfect guide for beginners to get acquainted with a variety of ways to heal the energy of your system. Some of the methods you will learn include yoga, meditation, mindfulness and how to use crystals for chakra cleansing and why they are so very important to the process.

Well, this book explains that whole process and how healing your chakras might help you need the doctor less and your own healing medicine more.

Chakras for Beginners will help you attain all of the information that you need to get started on your own personal healing journey. There are so many layers to the self and wanting to discover more about your unique life-force and vibrational frequency is a perfect beginning to tapping into the 'YOU' you have always wanted to be. Experience is not necessary or required in the field of chakra healing in order to reap the benefits of connecting to your energetic centers.

You and your body know so much more than you might think, and listening to the communication your body sends to you through your chakras is part of the pleasure of uniting with your own healing process. I hope you will enjoy taking this journey together and if you are ready to explore the intricacies of your beautiful light and vibration, then let's begin the colorful road trip through the chakras and give you all the resources you need to balance, cleanse, rejuvenate and live the life of abundance you have always wanted!

Chapter 1: A Brief History on Chakras

Since the popularization of yoga as a fitness technique, the word "chakra" has become something of a household term. Unfortunately, the word has also lost quite a bit of its original meaning, since many yoga instructors and enthusiasts fail to truly understand where the concept comes from.

This lack of knowledge on the origins of chakras is the main reason for widespread misinformation on what they exactly are and how they truly work in the body. That's why it's important to firstly develop an understanding of the historical background of these powerful energy centers to properly grasp their truth.

1*st* Thing you need to know…
They Originated In India

The origins of chakras can be traced back to prehistoric India at around 1500 to 500 BC.

Back then, they were documented in an old text called the "Vedas." This ancient collection of information contained some of the oldest scriptures, hymns, liturgical material, and mythological accounts of the Hindu religion.

In Hindu belief, the Vedas were created by Brahma - the first of three gods in the Hindu trimurti. Brahma inspired *rishis* with the knowledge and wisdom they needed in order to write the Vedas, and that's how the ancient text came to be.

The original Vedas revealed information about *"cakravartin"*, which directly translates in to the word wheel. They are referred to as wheels due to their association with a vortex of spinning energy.

2*nd* Thing you need to know...
There are More Than Just 7

Believe it or not, there are actually **88,000 chakras** distributed throughout your body. These energy centers are present over every inch of your skin and inside your system. In some practices, it's said that these chakras are interconnected.

For instance, reflexology – a popular alternative medicine - claims that manipulation of various points on the palms and soles of the feet can relieve ailments throughout other parts of the body. These "pressure points" are said to be energy centers where small collections of spiritual energy are concentrated.

Since they were first discovered however, 7 of the 88,000 chakras were given primary importance. These

7 chakras - aligned along the area of the spine were said to be the most powerful concentrations of energy throughout the body. Tapping into these centers would produce the most pronounced effects on the system, making them of utmost importance to Hindu believers and yogis.

3rd Thing you need to know…
They Tie In Closely With Yoga

One of the reasons why chakras have become particularly well-known today is because of the popularization of yoga as a fitness routine. Unbeknownst to modern yoga practitioners though, the original use of yoga was far less for flexibility and physical fitness.

The origins of yoga are fairly unclear since the practice was passed down through oral storytelling. Some of the earliest information on yoga was transcribed on leaves which were destroyed and lost just a few years after they were written.

What we do know, however, is that yoga dates back over 5,000 years. According to some scholars, the practice was used by early Hindu believers as a way of tying their physical self to their spiritual facet.

The information shared in the ancient Vedas gave them an understanding of their gods as well as their power over the lives of believers. Practicing yoga helped attune their physical bodies with their spirit through energy management, and made it possible for them to "reach" the gods.

The history of chakras is extensive; however, these three facts are the perfect introduction to help guide you towards the correct management of these intricate energy centers.

Chapter 2: Basic Chakra Truths

Those who are not necessarily spiritually inclined and even those who are do not always realize that their moods, amounts of energy, and motivation are connected to their chakras. A person who feels unmotivated, unsocial, and rather sluggish one morning at work can attribute this to a misalignment and/or weakness of chakra. It may even be the feeling of being surrounded by the negative energies of the managers and other coworkers. Again, one does not have to be super-spiritual in order to acknowledge, understand, and learn about chakras.

The concept of chakras was first discovered by Hindus in the 7th century BCE. They discovered the different energy points of the human body and that the soul can be found in different parts of it. They included these concepts in their sacred writ called the Upanishads. The Goddess Shri Lalita, who is said to reside in Mount Meru, is the deity often depicted in the pictures that'd you'd see of a woman's form colored in chakra points. She also represents the junction of both masculine and feminine energies in addition to the concept of all powers from different parts of the body working together.

Keeping Chakra Alignment

If one chakra is out of whack, then all the chakras are misaligned and negatively affected since they must all work together to keep the energy flowing throughout the body. You must learn to keep them all under control even if one chakra is more affected than another.

Once you know how to keep all your chakras under control and keep them unblocked, then energy flows freely. Hence, you will feel more motivated, driven and even more pleasantly social towards others. It is not difficult to learn to control your chakras, but it does take some hard work and commitment to keep the good energy flowing inside of you. Not only is this important in keeping yourself focused on everyday life and tasks, but also in keeping yourself in good health. Poor health and focus never go hand-in-hand. Once you get the hang of keeping your chakras aligned, you'll notice your life becoming much easier. Too much energy in one chakra can be just as bad as insufficient energies in another. For instance, if you open your red chakra too much, you may end up wearing yourself rather thin if you take on more tasks at a time than you should. You, then, most likely would not have enough energy and focus to complete all of these tasks properly and successfully or at all. If it's open enough to work properly, then you have enough sense to take on only as many tasks as your current energy allows so that they can be done properly and on time.

Homes of the Soul

The Brahma Upanishads talk about four main places in the body where the soul stays: head (the state beyond the physical human experience), heart (dreamless sleep), throat (dreaming), and navel (waking life). On the other hand, the Yogattava Upanishads believe that the body parts are linked to the main elements of earth, fire, air, and water. When one says they see an aura around someone, referring to a color, the color represents a person's current energy and vibration state. For instance, if you are currently experiencing constant sadness throughout the day, which is obviously natural and understandable, sometimes that energy can be transferred to another person and cause them to also feel low and sad, which in turn can hinder their daily activities as well.

However, if you're in a room filled with cheerful people that positive energy can transmit into you, leaving you in a happy, cheerful mood, in turn priming you to transmit said energy to others as well.

Wheels and the Sun

Wheels and the sun are two symbolisms associated with chakras. Wheels represent a constant flow, be it as part of an automobile or a water wheel. Meanwhile, the sun symbolizes order and balance, which are the main sources to keep our energies flowing, as the sun gives us energy as well. In fact, the word chakra means "wheel of light".

Chakras can sometimes become completely damaged, but this does not have to mean a permanent state, so long as you understand and acknowledge that they are in your body.

Again, all energies, negative and positive, will have an overall effect on your health. If a person is in a constant state of anger or sadness, they will be more susceptible to falling into poor health not only physically but also emotionally, and in some cases even mentally.

Misaligned or imbalanced chakras are equal to chemical imbalances, all of which can cause sudden mood swings. All you need to do is learn how your chakra points work and you will soon be on your way to a more stable emotional state.

The Body's Chakras and their States

Your body has a total of ten chakras: seven main ones and an additional three that don't come around very often. You shouldn't focus as much on the three additional ones though, because the seven main ones are usually the most affected by your moods and energy levels.

A chakra is always in one of these three states: open, blocked or sealed. When a chakra is open, it radiates the most energy and absorbs the most healing and alleviation from pain, illness, or other negative feeling or state. However, the only way to receive any form of healing from alternative practices is if the chakra is fully open.

A sealed chakra is not to be confused with a blocked chakra. In fact, a sealed chakra is actually a form of protection from negativities entering inside of you. Finally, a blocked chakra is an unhealthy chakra, as you are most susceptible to absorbing negative energies and a lack of flow of positive energies.

The Earth Star Chakra

The Earth Star chakra connects you to the Earth's elemental energies, keeping you more rational, logical, and focused instead of acting or speaking before thinking. These color auras are black, maroon and silver, and the best gemstones to use with this chakra point, often beneath your feet, are hematite, garnet, tiger's eye, and onyx.

Onyx and hematite are considered the go-to gemstones for blocking out negative energies. Earth star chakras just goes to show that the more grounded you are in your everyday life and conscious decision making, the more enjoyable life becomes. Conversely, when this chakra is blocked, you are more susceptible to depression, lack of interest in connecting with others and loss of motivation to do anything.

The Root Chakra

The root chakra, represented by the color red, is responsible for your family and survival aspects, in addition to how well you work and/or socialize within groups. Its point is at the tailbone of the spine and is believed to be the "root" of all chakras, hence its name.

In terms of physical health, when the root chakra is opened, your skeletal and circulatory systems are more likely to be healed, as well as your legs, feet, hips, and parts of the excretory system. The proper stones to use should be in the red and black family, such as obsidian, bloodstone, ruby, garnet, red jasper and red quartz. Keep this chakra balanced and you will see that you will work better with others and use rational-thinking to help out groups of people when need be, especially when problems arise.

The Sacral Chakra

This chakra point is found in the lower abdominal area. It is in charge of a person's sense of desire for adventure and connection with other people, as well as sense of pleasure, wealth (not necessarily in terms of finances) and sexuality, especially when it comes to understanding your partner's needs and desires.

Other concepts relevant to the sacral chakra are creativity and fiscal responsibility. Its color aura is orange, and the gemstones associated with keeping the sacral open are coral, carnelian, and amber. With these gems, you will feel motivated to finish your projects, especially creative ones, properly and in a timely (but not rushed) manner. You will also have the ability to better understand someone's feelings, as well as your own.

When the sacral chakra is blocked, you will be more susceptible to moodiness and lack of sexual desire or pleasure.

The Solar Plexus Chakra

The solar plexus chakra (also called navel chakra) is found in the upper abdominal area and when open, allows you to be in control of your own life, with confidence and no fears, while keeping your self-esteem high. Your confidence and self-respect, however, will not be limited to yourself—you will have faith in others too, albeit in a rational, reasonable sense.

The color aura is yellow, and the right stones to use, especially when you have illnesses and digestive discomfort are gold topaz, citrine, amber, gold calcite or any other stone in the yellow/gold family.

Any negative energies associated with this chakra are lack of self-worth and no sense of real self.

The Heart Chakra

The heart chakra deals with love, and not just in a romantic sense but also an overall compassionate one. It allows you to be loving and in a state of joy and peace, which in turn will allow you the ability and desire to heal others when they are sad and/or in some form of pain, be it physical or emotional. It also allows you to be charitable to the less fortunate.

The heart chakra's colors are green and pink and the appropriate stones to use would be: rose quartz, moss agate, emerald, jade, and aventurine.

Keep this chakra open in order to keep your respiratory system healthy and functioning properly. Also, remember that love and compassion, even the smallest gestures, will go a long way.

The Thymus Chakra

The thymus chakra is similar to the heart chakra, as far as unconditional love and compassion are concerned, only that there are more concepts involved. The thymus, located between your throat and your heart, is more in charge of allowing you to be accepting of others no matter what and without judgment. The thymus is also in charge of the endocrine system, which deals with growth, but not solely in a physical sense.

The colors associated with the thymus are green, purple and aqua. The appropriate and best stones to use are lapis lazuli, aquamarine, and turquoise.

When this chakra is blocked, you lose your ability to understand and accept others. Moreover, it becomes harder for you to show real love towards people and to accept any advice they would have to help you grow, particularly in a spiritual sense. You would also lack the ability to have lucid dreams or even good dreams for that matter.

The Throat Chakra

When the throat chakra is opened, you are able to better communicate and express your emotions to others, especially in a clearer, more confident manner while still being respectful. You also have an increased sense of creativity and can make rational decisions.

Located in the throat, it is responsible for bringing out all of your soul's true feelings. Hence, you'd be capable of hearing and communicating with spirits. Its color is a light blue hue. The gemstones you'll need to keep this chakra healthy are: sodalite, aquamarine, lapis lazuli, and turquoise.

When this chakra is blocked, any body part related to the mouth and throat will be negatively affected, as well as your overall intellectualism and curiosity.

The Third Eye Chakra

Located at the forehead, the third eye chakra helps you to "think outside the box", think for yourself, and at the same time, hinder shortsightedness or narrow-mindedness when it comes to others' viewpoints and inputs. Although this chakra allows you some form of psychic ability and communication with spirits (even the ability of astral projection), keep in mind that there is still a power higher than yourself.

You will find the third eye chakra in the center of your forehead. Think of the colors violet or a very dark blue with this chakra. With that being said, the gemstones amethyst, lapis lazuli, and fluorite are most effective here.

The nervous system is associated with this chakra, so in order to keep the third eye open, make sure you are mentally stable and that all five of your senses are working properly. When this chakra is weakened, you quickly lose interest in things and activities that once excited you, and you criticize others and yourself far too much. You would also experience major creative locks.

The Crown Chakra

This chakra connects you with the spiritual world and enhances your awareness of it even more than you imagined in addition to aiding you to enlightenment. It enables you to live in the moment with no worries or regrets because your mind is in a clear state. However, when this chakra is blocked, you will be unable to let go of past hardships and issues and are more likely to influence you to become depressed and narrow-minded.

The chakra point here is at the very top of your head, and its colors are white, purple and gold. If your brain and spine hurt, use selenite and clear quartz for healing.

Keep in mind that this is the most important chakra of all, so be sure to take extra care, as it can affect your other chakras, both negatively and positively.

The Soul Star Chakra

The soul star chakra represents the light that is found in all the other chakras. It also allows you to connect with spirits and be in tune with your soul to completely understand it, as well as the good things that the universe and life have in store for you. Located just above your head, the best gemstones for this chakra are Lemurian seeds and selenite. Meanwhile, the aura color is white.

Chapter 3: Guided Chakra Meditation for Beginners

Chakra meditation probably resembles a range of relaxation techniques with the express purpose of bringing balance, relaxation and well-being to each of your seven chakras.

To understand chakra meditation, it is necessary to understand the nature of the chakras in more detail. First we must deal with the distribution of life force energy. The universe is not only spreading this energy to Earth, but through each of us through our glands and organs. This energy is essential for all of us to stay balanced and healthy.

This energy passes through each of your seven chakras and merges at these points. As a result, each chakra is closely linked to every other chakra. To achieve optimal well-being, you must consider all chakras holistically.

Through meditation it is possible to achieve the total balance of your chakras. As a result, you enter a state of total emotional and physical well-being. This is the goal!

It doesn't take a lot of dedication to fit meditation into your life. Even meditating just 20 minutes a day twice a day has shown proven health benefits. You do not have to dedicate your life to the study of chakra healing to reap the benefits of meditation.

The most important thing to keep in mind during chakra meditation is that you want to target your blocked chakras. As a result of this meditation, you want to identify and open each of your blocked or overactive chakras.

The goal is to learn to control the energy that flows through each of our chakras to ensure proper balance. Keep in mind that focusing on just one chakra is often a counterproductive experience because the chakras are so closely linked. For the time being we are meditating them all as a whole unit. In chapter 7 we begin to explain how to meditate on each chakra individually.

To start:

The first step is to find a quiet place where you will not be disturbed during your meditation session. You want to make sure this place is calm and quiet. We recommend taking at least half an hour for this meditation, although you can divide the time throughout the day if that works better for you.

You want to sit comfortably on the floor and fold your legs in front of you. Feel free to use a pillow if you would otherwise find the position uncomfortable. You need to make sure your back is straight, but not stressed. Your hands will drop limp on your knees.

For starters, just sit in silence for a few minutes. You want to breathe deeply and evenly. It is important to rid your mind of negative emotions, especially anger and worry. These will interfere with your meditation and the chakra healing process. You want to be able to fully focus on each of the chakras.

You should feel the tension start to flow from your body. Pay attention and focus on each of the sensations you will feel.

It can be difficult for you to relax and clear your head. This makes perfect sense. In our busy, modern world, it is almost impossible to find the time for this type of exercise

Lake. Simply put, most of us are no longer in practice when it comes to clarifying our minds.

The best way to get through this is to practice. It may feel a little strange or uncomfortable at first. You empty your mind as if you were emptying a jug of water; that makes it easy to be filled with something else. But by practicing you will feel like you are clearing your head.

Here are some tips for getting a clear mind:

- Concentrate on your breathing. Inhale deeply through your nose, count to two and then exhale slowly through your mouth for twice as long as you inhale. Keep your breathing smooth without holding your breath. Make sure you breathe deeply - you want to check if you are using your diaphragm by putting your hand on your stomach. If you use your diaphragm correctly, you will feel your stomach moving outward as you inhale and going in as you exhale. You want to breathe this way to relax, not take shallow or deep breaths.

Close your eyes. This makes it easier for you to start your visualizations.

During this process you go through all seven chakras. For starters, start at the coccyx with the Root Chakra. You want to visualize this as a red light that glows and spins in the center of the spot you are visualizing. Make sure you feel it move in time with your breath.

Then shift your attention to the Sacral Chakra at the pelvis. You want to visualize this as an orange light that lights up and rotates in the center of the spot you are visualizing. Make sure you feel it move in time with your breath.

Then go to the Navel Chakra at the navel. You want to visualize this as a yellow light that glows and spins in the center of the spot you are visualizing. Make sure you feel it move in time with your breath.

Fourth, you want to go to the Heart Chakra. You want to visualize this as a green light glowing and rotating in the center of the spot you are visualizing. Make sure you feel it move in time with your breath. Make sure to take the time to acknowledge the progress of Earth to Heaven.

Fifth, travel to the throat chakra at the bottom of the throat. You want to visualize this as a blue light that glows and spins in the center of the spot you are visualizing. Make sure you feel it move in time with your breath.

Sixth, go to the Third Eye Chakra, which is located in the center of your eyebrows. This is not the in-depth process for opening your third eye, which will be described later. Instead, just visualize this as an indigo light glowing and rotating in the center of the spot you are visualizing. Make sure you feel it move in time with your breath.

Finally, finish with the crown chakra, which you can find at the top of your head. You want to visualize this as a violent or indigo light that glows and rotates in the center of the spot you are visualizing. Make sure you feel it move in time with your breath.

That ends your chakra meditation session. By practicing, you will gain more control and understanding of the energy that permeates each of these chakras. This is an essential step in your chakra healing development.

Common mistakes

When we start, it is easy for all of us to make these mistakes when trying to build a good chakra meditation routine. Just because they're easy to do doesn't mean you should do them.

1. Get started with a daily meditation routine.

It is very common for people, even those with a great interest in chakra healing and energy, to start meditating and then walk away and drop their routine. In this way, meditation is just like exercise. It's easy to go to the library and read any fitness you can get, but you won't see any real change until you actually hit the gym. No one else can do your meditation for you.

Stress doesn't take a day off in your life. It is important that you continue to follow these healthy meditation practices to stay healthy in your daily life.

That is why you never want to take a day off for your meditation practice. If your life allows, meditate a few minutes at a time two or three times a day. For example, if it is too much to meditate for 30 minutes at a time, do three 10-minute sessions a day; once in the morning when you wake up, once in the afternoon for lunch and once just before going to bed.

This is the biggest mistake new meditators make and never actually start their practice. It's easy to come up with problems that prevent you from meditating, but the reality is that there is one solution: to get started now.

2. Fall asleep

We are all busy working and with our lives. Often the only free moments we have for late night meditation are close to bedtime. You try to meditate as well as possible, but soon notice that you have fallen asleep. This can be crazy and frustrating because you don't see results of what you do, especially when it is hard to find another way to do it.

Well, if it happens that you go to sleep while you meditate, consider it a good sign of positive and healthy behavior. It is never good to get angry with yourself. Instead, consider it a sign that something is going well. It is normal to fall asleep because you are tired after the day's work. Instead of being angry, be happy that you could fall asleep without stress.

Even a few minutes of meditation techniques and focusing on the chakras before bed is a good start. The next morning you can then wake up and continue meditating where you left off. And this time you can meditate successfully, which will make you feel relaxed and give you the tools to get through the day.

3. Finding it difficult to hold the focus

Many beginners think that the secret of meditation lies in completely emptying the mind. They imagine that you don't want to think of anything at all. However, this is disinformation, because it is simply not possible to completely empty your mind and not think about anything.

If you can't concentrate while starting your meditation, don't feel bad. The focus you associate with experienced meditation professionals is the result of consistent and long-lasting meditation practice.

If your thoughts start to become unfocused while meditating, don't resist them. Instead, you just want to notice them and focus on your breathing and chakra again without judging yourself. As you meditate more often and more consistently, you will find it easier to control your focus.

4. Not preparing your meditation environment:

Once you have established a routine for your daily meditation practice, you should focus on creating a good environment that will make daily practice easier. You may wonder what this means to you. You should at least focus on the following:

- Set aside a place in your house where you can meditate freely. This space should be quiet and you should only use it for meditation or other spiritual exercises, if possible.

- You want to find something like a pillow or mat to help you sit in your meditation room. It is also good to set a chair aside for this.

- Place a stopwatch or other convenient time telling device where it is not too disturbing.
- All of these steps are very important. It is very likely that when you first decide to start meditation you will feel very inspired, but it probably will not be long. However, if you already have a meditation environment, it will become easier for you to maintain a routine that is consistent even during these "uninspired" periods. If everything is already arranged, chances are you will see the area ready for departure, sit down and start meditating.

5. Force yourself

If you are trying to meditate while in a noisy environment or if you have trouble concentrating your mind on one thing, then silence for meditation is both stressful and stressful. If that sounds like a situation you often find yourself in, it's best to just accept it.

But how is it possible to focus when surrounded by noise? The best thing to do is to choose a sound close to you that can hold your interest and focus on it. The longer you focus on this sound, the more it will help your meditation.

The best way to do this is to be aware of the sound and draw your attention to it. The more you practice with this, the easier it will be to feel comfortable in a noisy situation and still be able to meditate. You would think this is not possible, but it is really quite possible. When you become a more experienced practitioner of meditation, you will learn not only how to block the sounds around you, but also how to integrate them into your meditation.

So you should not think that you cannot meditate because you are not at home. Practice doing it wherever you have a chance. Next time you think you're going to fall off the meditation car, try practicing a bit even if you're traveling by public transport.

It will become easier for you to do this with practice. Once you get the hang of meditating where you are, it helps you reduce various negative mental illnesses and even improve pain tolerance.

6. Not setting a daily time for meditation:

Setting a clearly defined time for your meditation day in and day out is a very important factor in getting you trained to be consistent with your routine. While it is useful to be able to meditate anywhere, for consistency it is best to stick with one time. Our recommendation is to have this time early in the morning before everyday life becomes too distracting.

7. Set too high expectations for yourself

It can be a disaster for you to set expectations that are too high when you start your journey to learn to meditate. Like everything else in life, you will get frustrated and disappointed on some points.

Meditation is not just something you do. It is a way of life. It will become easier for you if you do it more often and more consistently over a long period of time.

What you can expect with these types of processes is noticeable, but gradual and incremental benefits. Certainly, you will notice more positive effects of meditation, the longer you do it and the more consistent you are with it. You want to balance your expectations as you begin your meditation journey.

What you will discover is that while you may not immediately see the benefits of chakra meditation, it is easier to see how your well-being has improved when you look back and reflect.

In our world, it is common for everyone to try to achieve the fastest results with the least effort on their part. But meditation is a much more subtle art, and it often takes a while to reap the benefits of this art. Just because nothing changes directly doesn't mean chakra healing is worth it. Often this is a marathon, not a sprint. So don't worry and just keep practicing with the tips above. Soon you will find yourself on your way to healing and enlightenment.

8. Giving up too easily

Just sitting and meditating on your chakras can be difficult, especially if you are not used to it. So it is perfectly understandable that you are struggling to develop the state of mind for effective meditation. We all start wrestling and wrestling, and there is no shame in that. The only mistake you can make is to give up and not get up the next day and try again. If you simply continue, you will notice that your mental capacity will increase. It has no choice. Exercising will eventually lead to greater results. So don't judge yourself hard and don't forget to keep going.

Remember that the key here is daily practice. You must first establish a routine for meditation to work for you.

9. You think meditation means sitting like a monk

You've probably seen an image of a monk meditating in a crossed leg pose. Perhaps you thought that all meditation was like this. However, this is not true. It is quite possible to meditate any position you like, especially sitting.

If you like to sit cross-legged, definitely do. However, if that doesn't work for you, just sit as you normally would and make sure you don't lean. The important thing is that you sit in a way that makes you comfortable.

Really, the trick is to meditate constantly no matter what position you decide to use. As you gain experience, you may want to see what you think about cross-legged. For most people who are not yet used to sitting in this position, it is not very comfortable at first, but often gets better with exercise.

10. Meditate only if you feel that everything is going well

You really want to make sure you make a habit of meditation, not something you do to everyone now and then. It is tempting to devote yourself to meditation only when you are feeling down. But this can hinder your progress in controlling your chakras.

Frankly, meditation is often more effective if you feel well. In this way, you can assess your well-being and effectively balance your chakras so that you are ready when life takes a turn.

Chapter 4: The benefit of the different chakras

The chakras are important for so many different parts of your body. They are going to help you to feel good when they are all in alignment. But when the chakras stop working the way that they should, you will find that it can be frustrating. When one chakra gets out of line, it isn't going to take too much longer before all of the chakras start to fail as well. You need to have all of the chakras lined up properly to ensure that you are getting all the benefits that you are looking for. Before you can work on increasing how well your chakras work, you need to know more about how all of the chakras work and why you would want to help them to get better. Here are some of the benefits that you can get when it comes to working with your chakras.

The Root Chakra

The first chakra to look at is the root chakra. This chakra is in charge of your foundation and can help you to feel grounded in reality. You will be able to find this chakra near the base of the spine, kind of near the tailbone area. When the root chakra is working properly, you will be able to feel grounded in reality and will feel pretty secure. But some of the emotional issues that are associated with the root chakra include survival issues like food, money and even financial independence.

Balancing the root or the base chakra will help the negative emotions in your body to become released. This helps you to gain more of the confidence that you are looking for and will encourage you to move forward with your life. A healthy root or base chakra can promote feelings of security and will help you to explore around in order to find your purpose and to achieve success. A root chakra that is balanced is also able to generate the flow of energy all over to the other chakras.

The Sacral Chakra

The sacral chakra is the one that is responsible for your connection and how well you are able to accept people who are different from you in your life. If you are having trouble trying out new things or meeting new people, there could be an issue with your sacral chakra. This one is going to be found in your lower abdomen and it is near the navel and a little bit in. You will feel really inspired and your life will just seem to flow. People will be attracted to some of your positive energy and many opportunities are going to start opening up for you. With a sacral chakra that is open, you will be able to live right now in the moment and to experience life to the fullest. You will also see that your stamina will increase, so many physical tasks will become easier.

The Solar Plexus Chakra

The solar plexus chakra is all about your confidence levels. If you feel that someone else is in charge of your life or you aren't able to make decisions for yourself, there could be an issue with the solar plexus chakra not working the right way. You will be able to find the solar plexus chakra in the upper stomach area. The emotional issues that are found in the solar plexus chakra will include self-esteem, self-confidence, and self-worth. When these are not working properly, it is hard to have the right amount of confidence to get things done during the day!

Being able to balance out the solar plexus chakra will allow you to feel a bit more centered in your spirit, body, and mind. You will be comfortable in your own skin and will be able to relax a bit more. The energy that comes from this chakra is going to permeate to some of the other chakras, which helps you to relieve some of the other psychological and physical disorders that are going on in your body. It will also allow you to become a bit more aware of your own energy and how to be more comfortable with your own decisions, such as following your intuition or your gut feelings.

The Heart Charka

The heart chakra is the one that is in charge of your ability to love. It is in charge of your feelings and how well you can feel compassion or not to others. If this one works well, you have the right emotions and love for the people in your life. When it is closed or blocked you may not feel love or concern for anyone and when it is too open, you feel emotions all of the time because they go overboard so much. You will be able to find the heart chakra right at the center of the chest, just a little bit above the heart. The emotional issues that are associated with the heart chakra include love, inner peace, and joy.

Balancing the heart chakra will help you to enhance your love for others as well as the love you feel for yourself. It allows you to have feelings of forgiveness, empathy, and compassion for the world around you. When this chakra is in good working order, you are able to connect with a world vision of the beauty around you just like a child would. With this chakra, harmony and peace are going to flourish in your relationships with yourself and with others.

The Throat Chakra

The throat chakra is the one that is in charge of your ability to communicate. When it is working properly, you know when the perfect circumstances are to speak up and talk to others. You can have good communication with others without being shy or talk too much. You will be able to find the throat chakra right at the throat. The emotional issues that are associated with the throat chakra include communication, self-expression of feelings and the truth when speaking to others.

Balancing out the throat chakra means that you are able to have more open communication and you don't have as many issues with expressing your feelings. You are also able to do these things without feeling judgment from others. It is going to promote more harmony and honesty with your actions and your feelings because you are able to live a life that is more free and authentic.

A throat chakra that is balanced is going to help you to be more successful with your communication inside of relationships and even at work. It can be really important if you are in a career that relies on self-expression and communication so working on this chakra can be very important in some circumstances.

The Third Eye Chakra

The third eye chakra is all about your ability to focus on and see the big picture of what is going on around you. When the third eye chakra is not working properly, it is hard to see the other side of arguments or of the story and you may become too focused on a little piece, holding onto it for dear life and getting into bad fights because you refuse to expand your thinking and look at the full picture. You will be able to find this chakra right on the forehead between the eyes and sometimes it is called the Brow Chakra. The emotional issues that are associated with this one include intuition, imagination, wisdom, and the ability to think and make decisions when it matters most.

When the third eye chakra is balanced well, you will find that your intuition is much stronger and even clearer and dream interpretation is fairly easy. You will also be able to form a deep connection with the universal plan of your life. When the third eye chakra is able to guide you through your universal plan, you will have a sense of more doors and possibilities opening up to you to help you reach your goals.

Benefits of Keeping Your Chakras Aligned

It is important to keep your chakras as balanced as possible for your good health. Your chakras are able to influence everything that you do and there are many things that can make them get unbalanced. From the little stresses that go on in your life to the illnesses that you may be dealing with, it is not uncommon to find that your chakras are not as aligned as they should be.

If you want to make sure that you are getting through the stress that comes with your modern day life and you want to ensure that you are able to stay happy and healthy, then it is really important that you learn how to align your chakras. There are many ways that you are able to balance those chakras and help you to live a holistic life, you just need to choose the one that works the best for your needs.

While too many people ignore their chakras and what they all entail, these chakras can be really important to your overall health and will help you to improve so many aspects of your personal life.

Chapter 5: Crystal healing for chakras

Crystals could definitely make your chakras better—especially if you know the right ones to use, and that's why you should never leave them behind. When crystals are placed directly over your chakras, they're able to give off divine healing energy that is released through the energy channels in your body. This then makes its way to the aura and changes it for the better.

So, which crystals should you be using, then? Here's what you have to keep in mind!

Root Chakra: Garnet

Garnet is deemed as the crystal of the Root Chakra. As it is in the color red, it works with the Root Chakra because it's able to keep you inspired and grounded. It helps you become motivated to achieve your goals in life and to make sure that you do your best whatever happens.

Since it is in the color of Red, you kind of get the sense that it's perfect for awakening the first of your chakras. When you start with this one, you get to make sure that everything else will flow smoothly.

With the help of Garnet, you'll be connected to the earth—you'd be able to fight addictions, material desires, and being attached to material things—because life is so much more than that.

Sacral Chakra: Carnelian

Next, you have Carnelian, which is known as the best crystal for the Sacral Chakra. It gives you a better understanding of humans, and human life, as a whole. More than that, it's also able to hone your creativity, give you emotional balance, and help you have unity with yourself and with the people around you.

It is important to tap into this chakra with the help of Carnelian so that you wouldn't have to feel like going against the flow brings you nothing, or that you won't feel like you are working for nothing. You'd always be at peace; you'd always be motivated.

Solar Plexus Chakra: Citrine

Solar Plexus is responsible for your connection with the astral world—and even with your own astral body. When it's out of balance, you might be hypersensitive and overly emotional.

With the help of Citrine, you would be able to neutralize the negative energies that you have in your life. You'd be able to protect yourself, and normalize mood swings so that you'd be more appreciative of what's going on in your life. More than that, you'd also be able to let abundance and success be in your mindset so that you'd be motivated to do your best to achieve what you want. It will end your depression and self-doubt—and help you become a much happier individual!

Heart Chakra: Aventurine

Green Aventurine is the best crystal for the heart chakra. It's always good to take care of the heart chakra because it's quite sensitive. When not given enough attention, it may cause you to feel separate from others. It prevents you from loving people unconditionally.

However, with the help of Aventurine, you can bring things back in order. You'd be able to set realistic goals and remind yourself to do your best in order for them to come true. It calms you down and prevents you from being angry or irritated at times when you have to remain composed. It heals circulation and helps you be more in touch with yourself, balancing male-female energy in the process. And, it also promotes compassion and empathy; it makes you understand you're not the only important person on earth; others matter, too.

Throat Chakra: Jolite

Jolite works with the throat chakra's main color of blue. It's a crystal that makes way for clear expression, and also keeps the lines of communication open. When it works with the chakra, it's able to help you figure out what's right for you, and tell you what you need to feel inside.

Jolite is able to help you speak from the mind and from the heart—and not just one of them at a time. It's able to help you speak your truth so that everything in your life would easily flow, and you'd be able to manifest positivity in any part of your life. Jolite is also able to promote leadership, power, self-confidence, and inner strength—helping you express yourself way better than before!

Third Eye Chakra: Amethyst

Not only is amethyst one of the most popular stones out there, but it's also essential for the improvement of the third eye chakra. You see, when the third eye chakra is out of balance, you will find it hard to meditate and attach yourself to your inner being. You might also have an irrational and intense fear of death and may make you depressed for quite a while.

As Amethyst is known as the stone of meditation, it has natural calming and healing qualities. It's able to bring harmony, peace, and calmness in your life. It also develops intuition, increases your attention, and helps you train your mind to make lucid dreaming possible. Aside from that, it gets rid of compulsive behaviors—and always makes you feel at peace with yourself, with the world, and all the other beings in it.

Crown Chakra: Rainbow Moonstone

And lastly, you have a rainbow moonstone for the crown chakra. The colors pink, purple, and white are predominant in the crown chakra, so it's just fitting that a colorful crystal is also used for it.

As the name suggests, people believe that the rainbow moonstone has some connections to the moon and that it has quite some magic of its own. The said magic allows you to open up your heart and mind to spiritual development and helps you appreciate spiritual experiences. It helps you forget the illusion of time and allows you to be calm while making use of ancient wisdom to rule over your life.

How to use the crystals

In order to use the crystals, make sure that you go to a quiet place and put your hands on the table. Keep the palms near one another, and ask a friend to go hold the crystals above your arms, and to point and rotate them. When you feel some tingling sensations, that's when you'd know that the healing energy of the crystals is working.

If the moment feels too overwhelming, feel free to take a break and put the crystals away a bit. Then, repeat the process again.

Meditation For The Sacral Chakra

Find a comfortable position while you are laying down preferably in the area that can become your meditational sacred place.

When you lay down, make sure to place a pillow under your head so you will not fall asleep, and another pillow, rolled-up preferably, under your knees to support your legs.

Your body will notice that it is not your usual sleeping position which will make you stay awake.

Turn off your phone and lock your doors to ensure that you will not get distracted.

When you lay down, strengthen your body, facing up and begin by breathing deeply. Keep your hands on your sides, with the palms facing upwards.

Start off by focusing your attention on the way your body moves as you inhale or exhale.

Relax your arms, legs, belly, and other parts of your body where you feel most tension in.

Gradually let your eyes close themselves, slowly and not forcefully.

Make sure to maintain balanced breathing, smooth, deep and slow.

Slowly begin to close your eyes gently, not forcefully.

Allow for your body to feel as if it's entering the deepest state of relaxation while the mind and the soul are wide awake.

Continue to breathe in and out, focusing on the way your chest rises and falls with every breath you take in.

If you find your mind wandering around, simply bring it back to your body and your attention to your breathing.

Take a couple of minutes to silence your mind, getting rid of any mental clutter and bringing the mind to a state of relaxation and meditation.

Once you relax your body, bring your awareness to how your stomach and organs expand as you breath in and out.

Feel any sensations or tingling inside where your sacral chakra is located at the lower abdomen, in your pelvic region.

Breathe slowly and deeply and try to notice any changes in the area of your focus.

Can you feel your pelvic organs pulsating or tingling as you breathe?

Continue to breathe deeply, relaxing your body in the process and observing your lower abdomen.

Bring your attention to the way you breathe in, as your organs are expanding and changing their shape when you inhale or exhale.

Imagine your kidneys, and other organs moving in your body slightly as if swaying from side to side.

Begin to call out to the universe and ask to resurface the life force energy from within you.

Ask for guidance and support while setting your intention to achieve constant healing within the sacral area, the gut, and the stomach.

Allow for that energy to resurface while imagining yourself glowing white color.

Feel the flow of energy throughout your body, resurfacing, recharging the body, and getting rid of any impurities.

Thank the energy within you as it constantly moves and tries its best to heal you physically, emotionally, and spiritually.

Form a Gassho with your hands and place them in front of you where your heart is.

Focus on centering the energy into your hands as you ask for guidance and healing from the Universe.

Once you've gathered energy white and pure energy within your hands, proceed by pressing them down onto your sacrum, the lower abdomen stomach area, that is a couple of inches below the belly button.

This is where the Sacral chakra resigns.

Allow that energy to hover in the sacral chakra, opening it and freeing its own energy.

Place your hands on the lower abdomen, skin to skin, and feel any sensations or movements through your hands.

Visualize the warmth radiating from both sides of the skin, picture an orange glow lighting up and warming up your hands.

You will start to feel tingling and movements in your lower abdomen.

Let it move all throughout your stomach and gut area, visualize receiving healing, improving your digestion, or even increasing your intuition, the gut feeling.

Lift your hands up and place them on your mind.

Visualize sending the healing energy into the mind, imagine opening it and balancing your emotions.

Think of all the negative energy simply letting go and moving on.

Replace those negative feelings that are letting themselves leave your body with those of happiness by thinking back to your happiest memories or about things that make you happy.

This will let the body experience its 'true' and happy state.

Imagine the light evolving and glowing brighter and brighter, radiating from your hands with the feeling of warmth and tingling sensations around that area whether you have physical contact with the skin or are simply allowing your hands to hover above.

Remove your hands and place them back on your lower stomach, the region that connects to feelings of enjoyment of living and happiness.

Allow for yourself to enjoy and live in this moment, notice the butterflies and the joyous feelings they give out in your stomach.

Each time you deeply inhale, bring that orange glow a tiny bit brighter and bigger.

Feel the creative and inspirational energy run through your veins.

Lay in that feeling for a few minutes before gently opening your eyes.

Breathe in the air around you and look around as you still feel that strong and bright energy.

Clear this area for about two to three minutes before placing one of your hands on your back, with the palms facing downwards.

Proceed to visualize further healing and opening of this chakra.

Allow for the energy to travel all around, to any tensions within the area and banishing any impurities.

Visualize cleansing and purifying the mind by healing and opening the Sacral chakra.

Hold your hands there for two to three minutes at most, resting your mind as you breathe in deeply and slowly.

Consider taking some time to gently massage the area to promote a healthy flow of energy, relaxation, and freedom of any tension.

If you choose to massage the area then make sure you do it clockwise for women and anticlockwise for men, or whichever way feels right to you.

Gently press three fingers, the index finger, the middle finger, and the ring finger against your exposes stomach.

Begin by gently applying pressure before massaging it in a circular way.

Proceed by breathing in deeply, holding in the breath for three seconds before letting go as you massage it.

Continue to visualize the orange healing energy swimming within the area that you touch, healing it in the process.

Slowly bring your attention back to your breathing, allowing for the energy to evenly spread back throughout your body while cleansing it and removing any impurities.

Rest for a minute before gently opening your eyes.

Allow yourself to lay in the feeling of being aware of your surroundings for a couple of minutes while reminding yourself of your pure intentions of healing yourself while cleansing the body with the energy.

Reflect on your meditation.

Did you receive any sensations or visions?

Often times during meditations especially with healing, the universe might speak through visions to hint something else that might be needed for healing, either physical or mental.

Breathe in the air around you and look around as you might be filled with strong and bright energy.

This new found energy might overwhelm you with a strong urge to create, so allow it to guide you in releasing the energy through creating some with inspiration.

Solar Plexus Chakra

The third chakra point is the solar plexus, it is also referred to as Manipura which means 'lustrous gem' and 'resplendent gem'.

Since the chakra is located in the upper abdomen, just a couple of inches above your belly button, it is known as chakra of intuition, or 'gut feeling' due to its location.

This chakra is the representation of one's willpower and the strong desire to achieve success.

It is also associated with wisdom, confidence, and the perception of who you are as a person.

The solar plexus is the origin of one's self-discipline and self-esteem that makes up a person as a whole.

It turns thoughts and goals into actions through willpower.

This chakra is associated with the color yellow which means energetic, cheerful, happiness, intellect, and encouragement.

When the solar plexus is imbalanced, the energy is either directed too much on the body or mind.

Physically, the solar plexus is responsible for the problems found within the muscular system, the cellular respiration, the nervous system, digestive system, blood sugar problems, hypertension, and gallbladder.

When this chakra is imbalanced emotionally, one will always suffer from migraines, changes in attitude, mood imbalance, and lack of motivation.

You will also begin to feel powerless in situations within your life, like losing control of everything that happens around you.

This will cause you to always be angry or lashing out to surrounding people, applying negative energy to the environment and influencing other people negatively.

Life will become a hassle rather than being filled with joy and living it to the fullest.

When balanced, one feels as if they have the power to accomplish any of their goals, this strong feeling is able to turn the thoughts into actions.

The balanced solar plexus chakra makes you feel full of energy, lively and gives you the ability to accomplish challenges.

You are confident in yourself and your power to follow through the difficulties that life throws at you while making sure that the mind stays in a calm, cheerful, and confident state.

Physically, the body is healthy and fit due to the fact that the solar plexus has all the control over the cellular respiration system within the body.

This makes sure that the body is in great condition and health.

The flow of energy throughout the body is balanced and strong, also aiding in the healing process of the body.

Emotionally, this chakra can ease the worries of the mind as well as releasing it and other negative feelings, maintaining the mind clear, healthy and well-balanced along with the body.

A balance in the solar plexus promotes strength, motivation, courage, and happiness in the body, mind, and soul, thus enabling this chakra to balance out the other major chakras.

When the solar plexus is underactive, it will disturb the flow of energy within the body.

You may start to experience a lack of control as well as a loss of purpose in life.

This often leads to a lot of emotional problems, self-destructive behavior, and self-doubt.

Underactive solar plexus makes one feel helpless, indecisive, grants a low-esteem, and a lack of confidence.

When the solar plexus is overactive, it means that the solar plexus has way too much energy in the region compared to other chakras.

You will experience issues in controlling people, yourself, and your environment.

Having control over your own life is good as long as it is not going overboard which an overactive solar plexus does.

When it is overactive, you will feel overwhelmed in energy that can overstimulate the system and tire the body out.

One will also become stubborn, aggressive, judgmental, and overcritical.

This chakra is best to be opened with meditation but adding certain changes in diet can also help greatly.

Eating yellow-based foods such as grains, yellow peppers, bananas, and corn, as well as other complex carbohydrate foods that are able to give you plenty of energy can help in the opening of the solar plexus.

However, you must avoid too many sugary foods seeing as the glucose is not natural.

Make sure to drink plenty of chamomile tea which is known to help clear the blockage of this chakra.

Decorating one's house with yellow flowers or wearing yellow clothing can help stimulate the solar plexus visually.

Meditation For The Solar Plexus Chakra

Begin with a light stretch, too relax the muscles for your meditation.

Stand up, and lift your hands up into the air as if you are reaching up to touch the sky.

Reach as far as you can while you take a deep breath in, holding the position and your breath for two seconds.

As you exhale, drop your hands to your sides, pulling the breath for another two seconds.

Lift your hands up again as you breathe in and drop them to your sides as you exhale.

Repeat at least three times before proceeding with the meditation.

Sit up in a comfortable position on the floor or on a chair in the room of your sacral chakra meditation healing practice.

Cross your legs, as you extend your spine nice and straight.

Lift your head up, as if you are balancing a book right on top.

Place your hands on your knees with the palms facing upwards.

Get rid of any distraction, by closing the windows, turning off your phone, and locking the doors.

Start off your meditation by breathing slowly and deeply while staring off into space.

Take as long as you need to relax your body, muscles, and adjust your mind from wandering around and gently allow for your eyes to slowly close.

Further bring your body to relaxation by focusing on and relaxing different parts of your body such as legs, stomach, chest, arms, shoulders, neck and head, as you move your focus along your body from top to bottom.

Take a couple of seconds to hold the image of yourself sitting up, while you are relaxing your body.

You can also direct your focus to how your chest and body rise taller as you breathe in or falls shorter as you breathe out.

Hold your attention on your breathing to ensure that your mind won't slip away.

By bringing your focus somewhere else except your mind, you are able to clear your thoughts from any worries of troubles.

Now that your body is close to its relaxed state and so is your mind, change the way you breathe to fit the opening of the solar plexus area.

Since the location of the chakra is on the lower part of your ribs, you will be using your chest to breath.

Inhale the air and expand your lungs, hold the breath for at least four seconds before exhaling through your mouth.

Visualize releasing any negativity through your exhale as your spine expands higher every time you breathe.

Focus on the way your chest rises and falls and don't let your mind wander away.

If it does, then gently bring your attention back to your attention to the movement of the spine.

Just like any other healing treatments, call on the Universe and ask to heal your solar plexus chakra.

Visualize channeling your energy and centering it on the palm of your hands.

Allow for the energy to resurface your body, as a white pure life force healing energy.

Let it hover all throughout your body for a minute, energizing it and gathering its strength.

Place your hands on the area above your belly button but below your heart.

You will be touching the lower part of your ribs.

You should place your hands next to each other and not overlapping each other.

Concentrate on making the energy flow through your hands and to the solar plexus.

Visualize it healing the chakra, clearing it of any blockage and releasing the negative emotions or negative tensions that could possibly affect the physical health of the body, imagine anything negative leaving through your mouth as you exhale.

When you are sitting down, start to connect and feel the coldness or warmth of the floor, the bed, or the ground beneath you.

Visualize the energy from the ground traveling up through your body, through your toes.

Imagine sucking in that energy that belongs to the earth.

Focus on this energy as it's moving up towards the location of the solar plexus which is in between your belly button and the bottom of your rib cage, also known as the upper abdomen.

With your hands still on the upper abdomen, imagine yellow glow forming and expanding in that area as all the energy begin connecting, rotating clockwise and getting larger every time you take a breath in.

Feel the warmth and sensation that the yellow light is providing and how it makes you feel emotional.

Keep your hands on that area for at least two to three minutes before moving on and placing your hands on the top of your knees, forming a mudra by touching both the thumb and the index finger together.

If you'd like, you can keep cleansing the area for longer than three minutes, however long you feel is necessary for your upper abdomen to heal.

Begin to imagine that you are sitting on top of a grassy hill, sitting right below the sun that is shinning right back down on you.

Your eyes are closed as your own sacral chakra begins to glow and react with the sun.

The energy tingling within your upper abdomen, experiencing healing and cleansing.

Focus your attention on the part of your body that you imagine is the warmest from the sun, such as the top of your head.

Yellow stimulates the feelings of joy and it also represents the solar plexus.

Feel and appreciate the warmth that you are receiving and accept the tingling sensations that are spreading through your body.

Then start to bring your attention inwards, notice how the ground beneath you feels like, is it cold or warm?

Can you feel any tingling or pulses through it?

What about the space above your head?

Does it feel like a whole universe is right above you just by feeling a little pressure on your head?

Freely lift your arms up towards the sky as you inhale and feel the astral world above you.

Picture a bright yellow flame at the tip of your fingers, feel as it connects through your hands and travels down to your upper abandonment where the solar plexus is located.

Breath out and lower your arms down to the ground.

Place your hands on the ground and feel the earth beneath you and the perfect balance of life and energy around you.

Inhale once more, raising your hands up towards the sky as if connecting your energy with the one with the sun.

Let the yellow glow travel down to you upper abandonment, clearing and opening that chakra point.

Notice what you are feeling during this moment, are you feel calm, balanced and happy?

Repeat the hand motions for a few minutes or however long you wish.

Place your hands back down on your knees, forming the mudra. Use the mantra 'ram' by saying it out loud physically.

This specific mantra vibrates the body and helps the negative energies flow out of the chakra and out of the body while leaving only positive and pure healing forces.

Mantras are just words that are said during meditations but it can also be used in practices to ensure that the body is cleared effectively.

Place one of your hands on your back, with the palm facing outwards while you repeat the same process of visualizing the yellow energy healing moving and releasing any tensions in the upper abdomen.

Take a minute to rest in the healing sensations.

To finish, place your hands back to the ground.

Breath in deeply with an open mind for a minute while bringing your awareness back to the physical world.

Imagine the room that you are in to help get back to your consciousness and the body.

Make an intention to express utmost gratitude to the Universe for guidance, your energy for healing you, and opening your solar plexus chakra.

Take another minute to simply breathe in deeply, in through your nose and out through your mouth.

Open your eyes slowly but do not move your body.

Look around you, take in the details of your room, stay in the moment for a few minutes while reflecting on the healing that you just achieved.

Heart Chakra

The fourth major chakra point is the heart chakra, also known as Anahata chakra that means 'unhurt'.

The context of the meaning connected to the heart chakra, when it is healthy and in balance, the heart and mind are not hurt.

The heart chakra connects to the mind, it is also the source of the deepest emotions such as unconditional love, compassion, passion, and joy.

The feelings of the heart are able to be expressed through the throat chakra and the mind, those deep feelings that are sometimes very hard to express verbally come from the heart.

Since the heart is the middle chakra, it connects the chakras below it and to the chakras above it.

The heart chakra is associated with the color green which represents prosperity, wealth in any aspect of one's life, health, and abundance.

This chakra can help heal both mental and physical issues.

The location of the heart chakra is right in the middle of the chest area.

When imbalanced, the heart experiences many negative emotions and negative energy in the body, mind, and the physical environment due to the fact that low vibrations attract other low vibration.

Negative thoughts and emotions can also cause the proper function of the body to fail.

Physically, the heart chakra is responsible for the problems found in the immune system, the circulatory system, respiratory system, muscle, and diaphragm.

Illnesses such as breast cancer, lung diseases, heart disease, allergies, asthma, high blood pressure, and other health problems revolving the heart chakra region.

Emotionally, this chakra deals with very deep emotions such as grief, anxiety, jealousy, hatred, loneliness, fear, and isolation, especially when the heart chakra is imbalanced.

You will always feel like you are stuck in the past or constantly thinking about the future, unable to focus on the present and what is really important at this time.

Negative feelings can cloud one's judgment, making one feel like they must always protect themselves when in fact there is no danger.

Negative emotions can also strongly impact the physical environment, causing separation, abandonment, and emotional abuse.

When in balance, you feel comfortable and healthy both physically, mentally, and spiritually.

When it is in balance, the body and mind are also at an equal with no worries, which satisfies one spiritually.

You are able to find forgiveness in your heart to those who hurt you in the past, which is also a great way to move on from that situation that left a mark on your heart.

Being stuck in the past doesn't help one focus on the present which is all life is about, enjoying and living in the moment.

The heart chakra grants compassion, peace, comfort, and gratitude for every little thing you have.

Physically, the heart is located within the heart chakra.

The heart is healthy, as well as the surrounding areas such as breasts, lungs, and ribs when the heart chakra is in balance.

It is also responsible for keeping us alive by promoting the beat of the heart and the blood circulation.

Emotionally, the heart chakra is known to be quite vulnerable but when it is in balance, one is able to experience the true meaning of happiness and what it is like to live their life filled with love and acceptance.

The mind is known to be in a very calm, confident, loving, and cheerful state.

However, that can also be the heart chakras undoing, being too cheerful and loving can sometimes backfire if it is given to the wrong people.

The underactive heart chakra revolves around the unhealthy distribution of the flow of energy within the body.

You will begin to experience an inability to forgive, forget, and move on with your life which will cause you to always be stuck in the past.

It can also prevent you from creating new relationships and opening your heart to more people.

This detaches you from the outside love as well as leaving you feeling withdrawn, isolated, critical of yourself and others.

The overactive heart chakra is distributing way too much energy, meaning that one can be giving away too much love and not leaving any for themselves.

This can leave you feeling emotionally drained and can affect your physical health.

An overactive heart chakra can lead you to feel a lack of discernment, especially in relationships as well as leave you feeling like you overexert yourself in terms of your personal life, this can make your relationships become toxic.

You will also find yourself feeling under control of your emotions and create a dependence on the personal relationships that you have with people rather than relying on yourself to be happy.

The overactive heart chakra can also cause a loss in personal boundaries, loss of identity, neglect, and always saying yes, even to things that can bring you pain.

Many times the main problems of having a blocked heart chakra revolve around a question, 'are you giving the same amount of love to yourself that you give to others' or 'are you putting yourself and your needs before anyone else'.

Many of those who have a blocked heart chakra either put other people before themselves or block their own heart from receiving love.

In order to open the heart chakra, one has to practice self-love and putting themselves before anyone else.

Your feelings and your own happiness are what matters most in the end.

Take some time to relax and gather your thoughts, follow the path which makes you the happiest self rather than pleasing and doing what other people want you to do.

Eating plenty of nutritious foods, especially those that are of green color, can help encourage the healing of the heart chakra.

Performing small acts of kindness such as smiling at a stranger or complimenting them can not only give out love but receive in the process.

No matter how much love one gives out, it will always find its way back to them in different shapes or sizes.

Opening your heart chakra will make you feel hopeful for the future, your relationships will strengthen with the people that you love and you will be able to attract more people into your life so place the stone above your heart or wear it as a necklace.

Meditation For The Heart Chakra

The key to healing the heart and chest area is through music.

Begin by picking a soft melody with gentle beats and sounds, no lyrics so you won't be able to sing along in your head.

It is scientifically proven that the right music can make you feel happier so make sure you find something that you feel a certain connection to.

Turn it on by a few bars that are soft enough to hear but not that loud, for example, 1/4 of the music bars.

Make sure that the melody is longer than ten minutes or on repeat.

Begin by laying down and relaxing comfortably.

Place a pillow under your head, and another under your knees for utmost comfort.

Leave your hands laying next to your body with the palms facing up.

Take a minute to focus and clear your mind by breathing in deeply.

Breathe in from your nose, hold the breath for two seconds and exhale through your mouth.

Continue this easy and simple breathing technique for a minute.

Inhale through the nose, and exhale through the mouth while setting a mental intention to relax your body as much as you can.

Proceed by gently closing your eyes and giving all of your attention to your chest area.

Use your lungs when you are breathing, instead of your stomach.

This means that when you breathe in, allow for your lungs to expand, moving around, filling up with oxygen.

Make sure that all of your attention is centered on your chest and the way it rises and falls or the way your body stretches upwards as you breathe in or shrinks as you breathe out.

Imagine that with every breath you take, you clear out the negativity within the chest, releasing it through the mouth, and allowing for yourself to let go of any tensions or impurities.

As you allow for your body to relax further and as you become more familiar with the deep breathing rhythm of your body, begin to listen carefully to the different tunes that you hear and try to focus on a specific one that stands out to you.

For example, if it's the sound of the bells you hear, then bring your focus there.

Try to push away any thoughts that might be emerging to the back of your head and relax while listening to that soft and quiet sound.

Take a moment to appreciate the music that you are hearing.

Observe how that melody makes you feel emotionally, are you feeling happiness and love in your heart, if so then continue by visualizing your heart fluttering as if it is opening up to love.

Think of flower petals emerging through your heart, floating around you ready to travel to your loved ones.

Keep in touch with your own emotion of love and connect it to the flower petals.

Think of a person close to you, a friend, a lover, or a family member, think of sending them those pink or green glowing petals filled with your love and empathy.

Wish them happiness and abundance through their life.

Picture those petals flowing to wherever they are now and connecting with their hearts.

Do this with two or three other people that you hold close to your heart.

Feel the warmth and tingling as more petals leave your heart and travel to your loved ones.

Let the energy gathered within your heart be released through your body, spread love throughout it and feel it within you.

Let the energy run freely up and down your spine through all the chakras, uniting them and growing your spiritual growth.

Proceed by making an intention to resurface the energy and asking the universe for guidance in this practice.

Focus on the white auric field surrounding your body, making you feel safe and comfortable.

You will begin to feel tingling sensations and warmth in different parts of your body.

Let the healing energy take its time resurfacing within your body and allow for it to center exactly where the heart is.

As you preformed the petal release exercise, the heart became more pure and positive, allowing for the energy to access it easier.

Place an intention to receive protection from anything negative in your life, negative events, negative emotions, and negative people.

This will help you feel safer and at ease from negativity.

Place another intention of receiving self-healing energy targeting the specific part of your body, the chest.

Allow for that energy to move from the heart to the shoulders and down to the palms of your hands, all connecting with one another.

Channel your energy and concentrate on centering it on your hands.

Allow the flow of white energy to resurface in your palms and glow a white and pure color.

Take a minute to just let all of the energy to catch up and gather in that area, healing the hands along the way.

Lift both of your hands and place them on your heart, one over the other.

Allow the energy to sink into your heart chakra and visualize the white-colored light changing into a bright green which is associated with the heart chakra.

Focus on feeling the beat of your heart against your hands, feel the pulsing vibrations underneath.

Rest in the moment as that green light sink in deeper into your chest.

Allow the energy to circulate and explore the chest area, going exactly where tensions are present.

Feel the tingling sensations throughout your body, smell the air around you as you take in deep breaths, hear the soft melody echoing in the room or against your ears, taste the freedom and the love life gives you and finally, although your eyes are closed, notice the glowing green light emerging through your heart.

Visualize the color glowing brighter and brighter as it opens your heart chakra to all the love and happiness that you deserve.

Think of the people who you care deeply for, imagine sending them your love and blessing to ensure that they are safe and happy with their life.

Think of different times when love was expressed and given to you, even the small things that made you happy still count!

Open yourself to healing within your heart.

Use the mantra 'yam' to help you open this chakra further.

Spend some time to opening your chakra, don't rush through the process but let your body heal its heart, either physically or emotionally.

Finish up by deeply breathing in and out through your mouth for a few minutes, just focusing on the music and the emotional feelings you receive from it.

The point of this meditation is to make you feel love to live, love for others around you, especially for yourself, and healing your chest area with positive and pure energy.

When you think you have finished, take some time for the energy to settle in within your body for a minute or two.

Allow for your eyes to slowly open, adjusting them to the light and the physical world around you.

Make sure to reflect on the meditation that you have just performed and the healing that you have received.

Proceed by doing something that makes you happy or something that you love.

Take some time to relax after the healing process, don't push yourself to do anything.

Stay at home, relax, take a hot bath, and let your body heal itself while the energy within your body is still present.

Throat Chakra

The fifth major chakra is the throat chakra that is also called Vishuddha.

Vishuddha means purification or very pure, and it signifies one having a pure mindset.

This connects to the throat chakra because, in order to have a pure mind, one must first be able to release the emotions and thoughts that happen within their mind through their throat chakra.

If the person is unable to find a way to release all the emotions, they can become bottled up in the mind, polluting it in the process.

The throat chakra is your ability to express yourself, the feelings inside the heart, and the thoughts inside the mind.

It is located within your thought region, representing the color blue which is associated with healing, peace, calmness, and content.

When the throat chakra is balanced, you are able to speak freely without no one or nothing stopping or preventing you.

You are able to express yourself and who you truly are, saying whatever is on your mind.

Those who are able to express themselves are also able to inspire others around them by speaking up and sharing their own opinion.

You know that people listen to you and are able to understand you.

Not holding or suppressing emotions and thoughts back will be able to clear your mind, returning it to its 'pure' state.

Physically, the area of the throat is healthy and in balance with the rest of the body.

Both the mental and psychological aspect of one's life is also in balance.

The throat chakra is accountable for the maturity and development of your body, especially the mouth, jaws teeth, vocal cords, throat, nose, and voice.

Emotionally, this chakra is associated with self-expression, letting go of the feelings that you were holding up from past situations that left a mark on your heart and mind.

Letting go and expressing yourself can be done through crafting, music, writing, and in many other ways.

It is important to let go and share your feelings instead of bottling them up inside of you.

When the throat chakra is blocked, you will have trouble expressing what it is that you think and feel, this will turn you into an isolated and shy person.

Physically, the throat chakra causes problems within the endocrine system, the metabolic system, sore throats, the hormones in the body, and the thyroid gland.

This chakra also causes many diseases such as hypothyroidism, laryngitis, chronic throat defects, autoimmune thyroiditis, and many others relating to the body's growth and throat area.

When this chakra is out of balance emotionally, you will suffer from feelings of low self-esteem, restriction, low self-love, isolation, and no self-expression, as well as feeling like no one is here to listen to what you have to say.

This can cause depression and anxiety.

An underactive throat chakra revolves around insecurity, introversion, and timidity, meaning that when the throat is blocked, one will struggle with speaking up and sharing their opinion which will detach them from their true selves.

Other factors such as fear of speaking, introversion, and small voice are the causes of an underactive throat chakra.

If the throat chakra is overactive, one will find themselves experiencing a lack of control over their own speech, meaning they will talk too much and say whatever is on their mind without considering the consequences of their speech.

Those with an overactive throat chakra will experience talking too much, criticizing yourself and others, struggles in relationships and feeling like no one understands what they are saying.

Other factors such as gossiping, arrogance, rudeness, condescending, and overly criticality is caused by the overactive throat chakra.

Since the color blue is associated with the throat chakra, drinking plenty of water can help open and balance the throat chakra.

Especially drinking warm water or warm herbal tea which can help release tensions within the throat and clear out negative energies.

Singing your favorite songs or humming to a tune is also considered as a way of speaking, speaking can help awaken and balance the chakra as well as releasing any negative energies or tensions within that area.

It is also scientifically proven that singing can raise up one's mood, meaning it can help heighten your vibrations.

Specific yoga poses that involve you stretching the muscles can also help balance out not only the throat chakra but other chakras too.

Consider leaving some spare time out to practice different yoga poses that relate to different chakras, it will help ensure that your chakras will become balanced and healthy.

An open throat chakra will make you speak clearly and will help you express yourself more freely.

Meditation For The Throat Chakra

Comfort is key, it is important to get comfortable when meditating so both your mind and body can relax and not disturb you through this process.

Start your meditation by getting comfortable, sit down with your legs crossed, your spine straight and reaching out as high as possible.

Make sure your head is not sulking, but nice straight and tall.

Your head should face the front as the chin is raised, imagine as if you are balancing a book on your head.

Form a mudra with your hands, an 'okay' or 'zero' look-a-like sign by uniting the thumb and the index finger together before placing it on top of your knees, the palm of your hand facing upwards.

Begin by taking a few minutes to relax your body and muscles, focus your attention on your breathing as your chest rises and falls.

Breathe in deeply, inhale through your nose and hold the breath for up to three seconds before exhaling it through the mouth and dragging it out for another three seconds.

Make sure that when you are breathing in and out that you expand your chest, instead of breathing through your stomach.

When you are using the chest, the spine extends and moves along with the breathing, this will enable the relaxation found within the body, as well as the throat region.

Feel the way your lungs expand inside of you as they are filled with the air around you, cleansing you, and getting both your mind and body ready for the pure energy of your life force energy.

The throat region is often linked with your voice, in other words, the awakening of the throat chakra can be used to heal both.

The purpose of this meditation is to take your worries away from your inability to speak up so try not to let the feelings of worry and anxiety take over, this is your time to let go of all the bad thoughts and let you be the person you are meant to be as well as healing the throat and shoulder region.

Take a few minutes to simply relax your muscles and the body as you breathe in.

Bring your attention to your breathing as you inhale and exhale to help calm the mind.

Try your best to not listen to your thoughts and the mental clutter that is going on inside your head.

Instead, bring your focus to yourself as a being in this big universe.

Imagine yourself to be one with the universe as the energy flows through your body.

Don't think about anything else that you have to do or things that might be bothering, instead focus on breathing through your chest, making the lungs expand as you breathe in.

Relax the different parts of your body including your throat and neck.

As you breathe in, feel how the air comes through your nostrils, to your throat, and into your lungs before coming back up.

It is clearing all the negative energy out when you inhale and lets it all go as you exhale.

Breath in deeply, form a rhythm of your body.

Begin the usual energy harnessing by calling out to the Universe, and making an intention to harness your life force energy.

Imagine a white light emitting from within your body, spreading all throughout.

Allow for your mind's goals to be clear by setting an intention to receive healing within the throat area and helping yourself speak up more and become more involved with the community through the healing found within the chakra.

Focus on centering your energy within your hands. Imagine the white light surrounding you, traveling all the way to your hands.

Let the energy catch up and gather there, forming a bright ball of light.

Lift your hands up and place them on your collar bone, one hand over the other.

Visualize the healing energy leaving your hands and sinking deep through your body and making its way to the center of the throat chakra.

While allowing the pure white energy to settle down, begin to visualize the color blue, think of the first emotion or thing that pops into your head.

Feel your body calming down and becoming more stable.

Then picture that color blue evolving through your throat, a gently blue glow expanding every time you inhale, merging together with the energy of the white.

The throat chakra represents the gateway between the heart and mind, you are able to freely speak what is on your mind and in your heart.

But just by thinking about it can bring forth feelings of worry, so imagine all that worry resurfacing and letting it go as you breath out.

This is your voice and your own opinions, you have the right to express what is really in your heart.

This is also a perfect time to release any stress or worries that you might have by simply bringing them back up to the surface and making an intention for the bright blue light to simply purify them.

Let go of anything that might be bothering you.

Feel the tingling and warmth sensations through your neck as they emerge and push you to want to open your mouth and speak whatever is on your mind.

Bring an intention forward to receive a physical healing, through the healing of the mind.

Visualize that glow becoming bigger and brighter for three to five minutes before drawing your attention back to your breathing.

While still holding your hands on that area, use the mantra 'ham' which can create vibrations that have the power to alter the flow of energy within the communication center.

Once you spend at least two to three minutes healing that part of your body, move your hands upward and extend the healing energy to your throat.

Hold your hands there for another brief two to three minutes before rotating and moving them to the back of your neck.

Allow for the white energy to sunk in right around the throat while releasing blue energy of the throat chakra, bringing in healing and relaxation to that area.

Visualize the tensions going away, the muscles relaxing.

Hold your hands against your throat for a minute before moving down towards your shoulders.

Allow for the blue light to intervene with the white, creating a light blue hue.

Let that healing energy work its magic, traveling and releasing any negative tensions within the shoulder area.

Rest that energy against the shoulders for a brief minute.

Allow for the energy to evenly spread throughout your body, returning back to its original state, this time more powerful.

Imagine the body relaxing and energizing itself as your life force energy returns back throughout your body, purifying along the way.

Continue to deeply breathe in and out for about a minute, simply resting in the newfound sensation.

Slowly bring your attention to your body, the way you breathe, or the weight that your body holds against the earth below you.

Open your eyes. Remain seated in complete silence for another minute, allow for the healing energy to further settle in while you take some time to reflect on your meditation.

To finish off the treatment, tell someone what is on your mind or sing your favorite songs before carrying on with your day.

Speaking, reading or singing can help heal the throat region much faster after the chakra healing that you have experienced.

Third Eye Chakra

The sixth major chakra is the third eye chakra, it is also known as Anja which means 'beyond wisdom'.

Just like its translation, the third eye relates to the concept of following your gut feeling, intuition, and the discovery of psychic ability, all of which are able to abandon critical and logical thinking.

The third eye is also known as the sixth sense, it is able to see things that are far beyond what the human five senses notice.

With the third eye, one is able to see into different worlds and see into what people are feeling, something that the physical eyes can't do.

Spiritual gifts emerge through the opening of the third eye since the third eye is known to connect one to the spiritual world and set one on their spiritual journey.

The third eye is located in between one's eyebrows, usually in the middle of the forehead, it is known to be the origin of foresight and intuition.

The third eye is also linked to the color purple which is associated with inner wisdom, power, intuition, and extrasensory perception.

When the third eye chakra is in balance, one has the power to not only see into their own soul and look for what they desire but also look into other people's desires and motives.

It is very hard to trick one with an open and balanced third eye chakra, they are able to see through a person and recognize their true motives due to the heightened intuition ability.

You also achieve a sense of confidence within your life as well as the knowledge of what you are here for the sole purpose of living.

You will also gain a strong sense of inner truth and resolving physical problems that will happen in your environment will become a piece of cake due to your intuition which will guide you through your life.

Since the opening of the third eye grants the person different psychic abilities, it also enables easier communication between higher beings, angels, and spirits as well as seeing into the future and seeing your past lives.

Physically, the body is in great shape and is healthy, everything, as well as the flow of energy, is in balance.

Since the third eye is one of the strongest chakras found within the body, it also can strongly affect the chakras below it, opening and cleansing them, bringing equality within the body.

The area that the third eye is located will function better, eyesight can improve, the brain will receive more knowledge, and many other related functions will increase.

Emotionally, the one who has an open third eye chakra is able to live their life freely and control their emotions to not affect the environment.

Clear thinking, decision making, awareness, seeing past lies, spiritual gifts, and a stable mindset is all thanks to an open third eye.

However, when the third eye chakra is blocked, one will start to doubt their own existence.

The questions of what is the purpose of life will constantly cloud one's judgment, refraining them from living their life to the fullest.

You will become disconnected with yourself, your environment, and other people.

Physically, the third eye is responsible for the endocrine system which affects the person's growth, metabolism, and maturity, it is also responsible for the hormonal imbalance as well as the sleep cycle, fatigue within the body, migraines, and headaches.

Emotionally, the blocked third eye causes anxiety, an emotional imbalance, a lack of understanding of reality, depression, and a feeling of always being lost or lacking something.

An underactive third eye chakra can negatively affect one's thinking, how they process information, concentration, motivation, and inspiration.

You will also become fearful of the things that you do not understand or the unknown.

You may experience a lack of intuition, believing everything people tell you, live in constant fear, and low self-esteem.

An overactive third eye chakra is able to overindulgence your mind and your imagination.

One will constantly be in a daydreaming state, with no focus on what is happening right now in the present moment within their environment.

When the third eye is giving off too much energy, you will start to feel mentally exhausted, and overwhelmed.

You may experience anxiety, become judgemental, overly analytical, experience indecisiveness, clouded vision, and judgment.

Yoga can help open the third eye chakra, specific yoga poses such as the eagle pose and the child pose is programmed to help open and balance this chakra.

Exercising and eating healthy can help all the chakras be balanced due to the release of negative energies, however, specific foods that aid the third eye are foods with high omega-3 fats such as sardines, walnuts, chia seeds, and salmon can help enhance the third eye.

When opening your third eye chakra, you will enhance your intuition and creative inspiration.

Meditation For The Third Eye Chakra

Begin by selecting a place where you will feel comfortable and undisturbed, so lock your doors and turn off your phone.

Put on some loose clothing so you will feel more comfortable and lower the lights if they appear to be too bright for you.

It is recommended that you lay down during this process but you can sit up if you want to, however, you might find it hard to hold yourself upward in a chair.

When laying down, remember to not place a pillow under your head, only under your knees.

You can use a blanket to keep you warm but make sure to leave your hands by your sides on top of the blanket.

Proceed by slowly closing your eyes, breathing in deeply.

Focus on your breathing, in with the nose and out through the mouth.

Allow yourself to become in tune with the moment that is happening right now.

Feel your arms and legs become more relaxed.

Breathe in once again and this time hold the breath for an instant before you let go through your mouth, feel yourself relax even further.

Each time you breathe in or out, notice how every second your body becomes more and more relaxed.

Bring your attention to whatever is beneath you, if it's the bed or the ground, feel yourself connect to that energy.

Imagine your own energy connecting to the ground, like roots of a tree extending right into it, convincing and intertwining with the energy of the earth.

Embrace it and let it travel through your spine, let go of any anxiety, fear or resistance that you might have.

Allow for the earth's energy to travel upwards, all the way to the top of your head.

Imagine branches and leaves sprouting from the top of your head. You are a tree now, in your visualization.

You are one with the earth and the universe.

Allow for the energy to sprout and grow, for the roots to extend all the way below you and the branches and leaves to grow above you, reaching towards the ceiling.

Allow for your energy to resurface by visualizing a white light emerging from within your body.

Let that light grow, growing brighter with every breath you take.

Center your energy to your palms.

Close your eyes and concentrate on visualizing a white light emerging and entering your palms.

Let the energy rest there for a brief minute, gathering and forming a bright bulb of light. the third eye, immediately lifting your spirits up.

Focus on transmitting the energy and getting rid of any tensions and blockages.

Visualize the third eye-opening, enhancing your intuition and other psychic abilities.

Lift your hands up and place them on your head, each hand on the side of your temples.

Continue breathing deeply and slowly as you focus on releasing that energy into your mind with the intention to achieve healing.

Draw your attention to the middle of your eyebrows, where the third chakra is located.

Feel the energy that has emerged from your temples, making its way into the center of your forehead, feel the tingling as it is opening and radiating indigo light in all directions.

Visualize both lights combining together.

It small and faint at first but it is growing with each deep breath you take.

Let go of any uncertainties as you let the light evolve within your head, healing any tensed areas that you might have.

This experience is natural and completely safe.

Let the indigo light purify your frequency and heighten it, drawing positive feelings and experiences towards you.

Just relax, stay calm, breathe deeply and allow the experience to happen.

Let the indigo light open in your forehead, sending the gently streams of its like in all directions, relaxing you in the process.

You will start to feel the tingling sensations on that point if not already.

Enable to relax your body further and further.

Feel your weight on the floor or the mattress if you are laying down become lighter and lighter as more light flows around and through your body.

Allow your mind to open by itself naturally and on its own, don't force healing to happen otherwise too much energy can backfire and not work.

Let go of any thoughts or worries that can cloud your mind and stop you from continuing with the process.

Don't think too much of what can happen but relax your body further and focus on that warm, tingling sensation between your brows.

Using your index finger place the finger down on the third eye chakra and start to massage it in a clockwise circulation for women and an anticlockwise circulation for males.

Don't stop the light from flowing through your body as you massage your third eye, releasing its energy and letting it join together with the energy of the chakra.

Allow for yourself to feel the energy flow through you as your chakra point is opening.

Breath in deeply and out through your mouth to clear and cleanse any negative feelings or energy within your body, this is only a pure experience.

You might begin to see visions in your mind or hear something calling.

Since this healing practice is located so close to the third eye chakra, it will naturally begin to heal it and opening it.

The third eye is known to see things that can't be seen with your physical eyes, don't stress over the newfound feelings that might erupt in your body.

Simply continue this very pure experience.

It might begin to feel as if your mind just naturally wandered away, or you are having a daydream but you are not making it all up, that is the energy of the guides that are helping you realize what else needs to be done.

Begin to say the mantra 'Ksham' out loud for another two to three minutes to encourage the healing energy.

Slowly bring your attention to your breathing and make an intention for the energy to fall back evenly throughout your body, purifying and cleansing it in the process.

Make an intention to return your energy and spread it out evenly across your body.

Take some time to simply stay in the feeling of being aware and conscious of your surroundings but at the same time remind yourself of your pure intentions of healing and cleansing your body with the help of the third eye chakra.

When you feel as if you have meditated long enough and that you are done, slowly bring your consciousness back to what is happening right now.

Feel how heavy your body is becoming as you are focusing back on what is happening right now, in this present time.

Become aware of your legs, arms, hands, and body.

Open your mouth and say 'I am fully present, here and now'.

Your voice might come off as if you haven't spoken in a long time.

Take another and final deep breath, holding it in for a minute before slowly opening your eyes.

Take a minute to simply rest while reflecting on your meditation.

Crown Chakra

The last seventh chakra is known as the crown chakra, it is the hardest one to open and balance.

The crown chakra is also known as Sahasrara which translates to 'thousand-petaled'.

The crown chakra is the conscious chakra, compared to all the other chakras below it.

It revolves around your own personal consciousness and the subconscious part of the person.

This chakra is also responsible for attracting the same level of vibrational beings or things into one's life.

Located at the top of your head, the crown chakra acts like a magnet, pulling things the same vibrational frequency as your body towards you, it also extends upwards towards the universe and connects you to the higher energies.

The color this chakra is associated with indigo which represents devotion, inner wisdom, intuition, self-responsibility, spirituality, and trust.

When the crown chakra is in balance, you will feel a deep connection to the universe, the higher power, and with yourself.

You will also begin to feel as if something or someone is watching over you, making sure that you are going towards the right direction and clearing up your path towards success by making sure you avoid the difficulties and bad things in life, that is if you vibrate on a high level.

This energy is looking after you understand exactly what you desire and is able to help you achieve your goals along the way.

You will begin to feel a deep and strong sense of gratitude towards not only the universe but to yourself as well.

Feelings such as appreciation and love to yourself, your environment, and others around you will feel at peace surrounded by happiness and the feelings of safety.

When good things happen, they are able to affect our emotional states which affect the vibration level and works to attract more good things into our lives.

It is not only important to understand that even if bad things happen, but there is also always a good side to them, a hidden lesson that the universe is teaching you and it is up to you to be able to understand it and connect it to your life.

When this chakra is balanced, you will feel like everything within your life is going by perfectly and smoothly that is because you understand that you control your own life and can shape your own future with the power of thoughts and high vibrations.

There are absolutely no fears, worries, or problems resigning within your mind and even if there is one, you are able to deal with it on a positive level that doesn't even affect your wellbeing, either mentally, physically, emotionally, or spiritually.

Physically, the crown chakra is responsible for not only the mind area of the body but the other chakras too.

The mind is able to not only cause illnesses but heal them too.

When the mind is in balance with the body, the chakras can feel the peace and begin to open up their pure energies.

Emotionally, the crown chakra is aligned with the body, mind, and spirit and promotes a healthy mindset.

When the crown chakra is blocked, then it is able to influence and block other chakras due to this incredible amount of energy found within the crown.

You will begin to feel disconnected from the higher power as well as your spiritual journey.

You will feel as if there are no 'angels' watching over you and that your life is going downhill.

Physically, the body will begin to always feel exhausted, out of energy, minor headaches, trouble in many of the body's systems, organs, and glands.

Many parts of the body like the nervous system, brain, pituitary gland, and many others will be affected by the imbalance. Illnesses like

Illnesses such as brain tumors, amnesia, migraines, and cognitive delusions are caused by the imbalance within the crown chakra.

Emotionally, you will be filled with feelings of isolation, loneliness, insignificance, and a lack of connection.

The feelings of anxiety, stress, depression, hysteria, and other mental illnesses are all the causes of the crown chakra due to its location.

Not only that but negative thoughts and feelings are able to damage the body physically too when there is too much energy, especially negative energy, directed in a specific location, it can not only overflow but temporary stop that part of the body from working.

You will also constantly be afraid of change which can put you in an environment that will cause your unhappiness.

The underactive crown chakra is when the crown is blocked, thus blocking other chakras and the proper function of the body.

When it is underactive, it can limit one's ability to let go of either of the past or any materialistic needs.

It will detach you from the world around you and lead to s spiritual malaise.

Not only will that but the relationships that you've built with other people be strongly influenced the negative way.

Other signs of an underactive crown chakra are mental fog, feeling of greed, lack of motivation, and lack of inspiration.

An overactive crown chakra gathers way too much energy in one place, it can cause a disconnection of the physical body, as well as an overwhelmed feeling due to the energy.

This will affect the physical body, giving headaches and migraines.

Other signs such as superiority, lack of empathy, and a sense of elitism are all caused by the overactive crown chakra.

If you drink many herbal teas, they are guaranteed to help reduce the blockage within the crown chakra by clearing and cleansing the body from negative energy and toxins.

While consuming specific indigo-colored foods such as eggplants or grapes, they are known to help the crown chakra balance itself out.

Once your crown chakra is open, you will feel a spiritual awakening.

This chakra is a pathway to all the other chakras which is why it can be the hardest to open for some people.

Meditation For The Crown Chakra

Begin by getting comfortable by sitting with your legs crossed, spine straight and shoulders back.

Place your hands on top of your knees forming the mudra, an 'okay' or 'zero' look-a-like hand gesture by allowing the index and the thumb finger on each hand touch, or just simply place your palms on your knees, making them face upwards.

You can even meditate outside in nature which can help you feel more connected with the world around you.

Start off by simply breathing deeply, form a rhythm with your breath as you inhale and exhale.

Inhale through your nose, hold the breath anywhere from two to three seconds before letting go through your mouth.

Make sure when exhaling you drag the breath out for another two to three seconds.

Relax your body, each part at a time, like your legs, arms, belly, shoulders, etc.

If you find your mind drifting away, focus on your chest rising with each breath you take and the way it fills and expands your lungs with oxygen, this way your mind will become more relaxed and will prevent unnecessary thoughts from emerging when you get further into the meditation.

Once you feel as if your mind is settled in, then focus on feeling the energy through the ground with each breath you inhale, you can sense it more and more.

Continue by bringing up that energy, make it travel up your spine, through all of the previous regions with your body, purifying and relaxing on the way.

Let it travel up your spine and fill your other chakras in with energy and finally let it travel to the last region, the crown of your head, located slightly above your head.

It signifies your subconscious and conscious mind which can affect the body spiritually, physically, and mentally.

Let that energy gather around like a faint ball of light, floating just above your head.

With the color white to signify purity and spiritual awakening, let that light connect you to the universe.

Picture the bright glow becomes bigger and brighter with each deep breath that you inhale.

Spend some time focusing on this magnificent ball of energy and light, observe how it makes you feel emotionally and physically.

Can you feel overwhelming energy radiating from that ball of light?

Or can you feel tingling sensations or warmth coming from above that area?

At this point in the meditation, you might start to forget about your physical body as you are connecting with that energy on a spiritual level.

Surround yourself with that light, imagine it flowing through your head into your third chakra, then to your throat chakra and so on until it reaches your root chakra.

Let it rest at each point for a few seconds before moving on to the next chakra point.

Make the energy come back up to the crown at the top of your head.

Let it rest there for a few minutes, glowing and warming up your head before it comes back down to the root chakra and then back up to the crown once more.

The energy should travel up and down three times.

Let the energy flow back through your body to the ground through the bottom of your spine or where your body touches the ground.

Observe any emotions that you might be feeling when the energy was moving up and down or when it left and merged with the ground.

Breathe in deeply for a minute, resting in the sensation of having all your chakras united and opened.

Set an intention to resurface the energy that is already there within your body, ready to be called to healing.

Allow the bright light of your energy to resurface, surrounding your body like an auric field.

Let the light warm your body, purifying your soul and removing any negative impurities that are the cause of all of your troubles and pains.

Center all of that energy into the palms of your hands.

Allow the energy to form a ball of bright and pure light.

Lift your hands upright in front of your chest and form them into a Gassho position, the national praying and gratitude gesture.

Draw your life force energy further into your hands and ask the Universe for guidance to be able to heal your mind, getting rid of any bad habits that need to be healed.

Channel the energy in your hands.

Lift your hands up as high as you can while still maintaining the Gassho position.

Hold the position for a couple of seconds before lowering your hands and placing them one over the other on top of your head, where the crown is.

Feel the tingling sensations and make an intention to open this chakra.

Hold the position for about three minutes before beginning to massage your head with your hands in a circular clockwise motion.

Visualize giving more healing energy to the crown and your subconscious while concentrating on opening the crown and healing the mind, body, and soul.

Get rid of any negative emotions that do not belong within your mind by simply making at the intention for them to vanish.

Breathe in through your nose and out through your mouth.

Move your attention to your breathing and imagine that with every breath that you take, the air inside your lungs travels to all different parts of your body that the mind controls, purifying it and granting it the energy it needs to do its day to day activities.

Proceed to heal for another three minutes.

As the energy heals the body, keep on breathing deeply as you begin to lightly say the mantra 'ohm' to help further intensify the healing energy.

Proceed to carry your attention back to the top of your head before slightly moving your hands lower to your temples, engaging with the third eye region for a minute while stimulating the flow of energy.

Return the energy to all of the body, cleansing and purifying it with its powerful energy.

With your eyes still closed, take a deep breath, hold it for five seconds before letting it go with your mouth.

Give your chest the attention that it needs to ensure that the mind is aware of what is going on around it.

Take a minute to let the energy settle down as you meditate normally, keeping your mind from slipping away.

Slowly begin to bring your awareness back into your body by noticing the weight that you have against the physical world before you open your eyes and stay put for another minute.

When the crown chakra is being opened, you might feel like your head is going to explode.

You might get some headaches because the energies are being drawn to you and everything else that is not important is being let go.

When the energy is released, you will feel tingling sensations throughout your body, as well as heat, electricity, and sparks.

Raise your vibrations by doing something that you enjoy and love deeply after the meditation.

Consider taking some time off to relax while letting the energy that you just experienced settle in and continue healing you and the body.

Chapter 6: Chakras Energy System- Living with Your Own Energy

Once you have accepted the power of your journey of self-discovery, you can begin to live your life every day with this understanding and connection to your chakras. We all have jobs, rent, bills, obligations, relationships, activities, and all manner of things that need taking care of in our lives. There are no rules for how you choose to live or how you incorporate your healing practices into your daily life; only you know the true answers to that. There are several things that can help you stay aligned in your chakras, however, that can be a great way for you to get started with empowering your journey.

As you begin to shift and heal your chakras, take into consideration how you are currently living your life. You may recall from Chapter 4 that there are a lot of significant ways that your chakras can be imbalanced, blocked, deficient and excessive. Some of those ways are:

- Excessive drugs, substances, alcohol
- Poor diet
- Lack of exercise
- Abusive or manipulative relationships

- Excessive television viewing, screen time, social media

- Dead end jobs that cause anxiety, depression, and stress

- Family issues

There are so many more ways that your chakras can collect energy that keeps you blocked and cloudy and in order to heal well, you will need to make some serious lifestyle changes. Before you get overly concerned about how that must occur, pay attention to why you are feeling that way in the first place. You may be excited to turn your life upside down and give yourself a new adventure toward the life you want. If you feel scared, worried, uncomfortable, skeptical or resistant to making any of the changes in lifestyle mentioned above, then you are in need of some serious energy clearing in some or all of your chakras.

The point of healing your energy is to help you align with your true purpose as a person in your life. How can you live your whole truth if you are unwell, unhappy, energetically imbalanced and suffering from significant blocks in your system?

Making the choice to clear your chakras is a big enough step in itself. No matter how long it takes you, even if it takes years, if you are committed to healing your chakras, then you will find the life you are looking for. Here are some of the ways you can promote life changes to help you heal and live with your own energy as your guide:

- Choose yourself first, before you choose others.

- Ask yourself how you are feeling whenever it feels right to do so. Keep a healthy, open communication with yourself, your feelings and your energy.

- Learn more about how you can open your chakras through yoga, breathing exercises, crystal therapies, acupuncture, massage therapy, Reiki and more.

- Take time in nature. Schedule time when you can be alone in the woods or on a hike.

- Practice oneness with yourself by being alone and tuning into your energy multiple times a day. Chakra check INS can be an excellent way to stay involved with your energy shifts.

- Take some new classes to awaken your chakras. You may find a ballet or dance class for your sacral chakra, or a painting class. You might find a writing class to open your throat chakra. You can take a class in pottery to connect you to your root and the earth. You could also start getting an education in the vocation you have always wanted to pursue but were too afraid to which will open and purge all of your chakras on some level.

- Bond with your personal space and make sure it feels right for your healing journey.

- Open up to loved ones about your experiences and let love in while you do so.

- Move to a new apartment or house in a neighborhood that feels safer or more affordable for your lifestyle needs.

- Change your job to something more like who you are, not what you think you have to be.

- Engage in healthier relationships and be willing to say goodbye to the ones that keep you stuck and away from healing yourself.

- Accept that your energy is always with you and a part of your life and is affected by everything you do, experience, choose and think.

All of these offerings are meant as guidance and support; a creative way for you to get started living with your own energy. Take your time moving forward. You don't have to change all at once. You will find that it happens naturally and slowly with your chakra healing experience and you won't have to think about it all that mush. Living with and accepting your energy offers it a chance to guide you. It is who you truly are and when you are cleansed, clear, purged, and unblocked in your chakras, your life can flow more freely and smoothly.

Living with your energy is a life practice and you are the one who will decide how to make all of the changes you need to make to have a healthy energetic life. Your chakras are ready for you to make the right decisions for you and will guide you forward, no matter what. Listen to your chakras and learn to live with your own energy.

Chapter 7: Some yoga exercises

In this chapter, we shall take a look at some of the yoga exercises that you can practice in order to balance your chakras.

Pranayama to activate your chakras

Pranayama is considered to be the most important of the various yoga exercises. Three minutes is the maximum amount of time a person can go without breathing, that's it. No one can survive without breathing. When you can keep your breathing under control, you will be able to ensure that your mind is fully focused. You will also notice that your body has managed to acquire a particular amount of balance as well. You will be able to maintain the energy and also the new found balance. Not just this but you will also discover that your chakra system has opened up and it is functioning in the manner that it is supposed to.

When you breathe properly, your body will be filled with sufficient oxygen. It is this oxygen that helps with the flow of energy in your body. Think about this from a scientific perspective. Only when you have got sufficient oxygen in the body will you be able to function properly and the same principle applies to the chakra system as well.

Reclining bound angle

This exercise is used for healing the Root Chakra. For practicing the reclining bound angle, you should sit up straight on a yoga mat. Then keep your feet stretched out in front of you, while your back is arched and your chin is tucked into your chest. You can either keep your hands to your sides or you can also place them on top of your thighs as well. Bend your knees and you will have to slowly draw your heels towards your pelvis. Once you have done this, you will have to press the soles of your feet together and stretch out your knees to the side, as far as you possibly can. Then lean backwards and transfer your weight by leaning onto your elbows. Keep lowering yourself onto the mat and you can make use of your hands to move slowly. Take a deep breath and move your hands into a prayer position over your head. Try to elongate your body by moving your buttocks into a convenient position. Let your body relax completely and slowly start bringing your knees to their original position once again. While performing this exercise, don't hold onto your breath, you need to keep breathing comfortably. Make sure that you don't hurt your ligaments while you are moving out of the position. Keep breathing slowly and move out of the position. Role onto your side and sit up comfortably. Ensure that your movements aren't jerky.

Child's Pose

This exercise can be made use of for healing different chakras. Mastering this chakra exercise will come in handy since you can reduce the amount of time that you would have usually spent on healing your chakras through all the different asanas. To start this exercise, you should kneel on your yoga mat. Keep your hands positioned on your thighs. Keep your back straight and lean back onto your heels. Now you should bend forward till your chest touches your thighs. You need to keep breathing comfortably while performing this exercise and also make sure that your forehead touches the floor. If you want some support while performing this exercise, then make use of your hands. You will have to curl your shoulders and then slowly move your hands towards your feet. Your palms should be facing upwards and when you think you are ready to come out of this position you should slowly move your arms, so that they are in front of your head. You should keep taking deep breaths while coming out of this position and you can support yourself while lifting yourself up from the position you are in. For transitioning into your initial pose, you should lift your back.

Cow Pose

If you want to concentrate on healing your sacral chakra, then this is the perfect pose for you. However, you really shouldn't perform this exercise if you have a knee or a back injury. For performing this exercise, you should start out by sitting straight on your yoga mat, keep your feet stretched out in front of you and your back arched upright while your chin is tucked into your chest. You can either keep your hands on your thighs or to your sides. Slightly bend your knees while keeping your feet flatly planted on the ground. Now, bring your left foot to rest underneath your right knee and slide it towards the outside of your right hip. Rest your right knee right above your left knee. Make sure that you aren't sitting unevenly. You should move your left hand towards the ceiling with the palm facing forward. Move your left hand towards your spine and your right hand towards your left hand, so that you are holding your hands. Now roll your shoulders and stay in this position for about a minute. Then slowly start moving your right hand away and lift your left hand up while holding it upwards. Slowly get back to your initial position with your hands by your sides. Relax and take a deep breath.

Camel Pose

This is probably one of the easiest poses to hold. You will need to ensure that you are flexible for performing this exercise. Start by kneeling on your yoga mat and place your hands on your hips. Your feet need to be resting on the map and start by slowly moving your spine towards your back. Bend backwards and you should place your hands on your feet. Stretch your neck a bit and elongate your spine.

Move your hands to your heels slowly. While you are moving out of this particular position, you should firstly move your hand slowly away from your feet so that you stay balanced. Then you can move your hands to your sides and raise your head. Stretch your back slowly, relax and breathe slowly.

Bridge Pose

This is the best-suited exercise when you are working on healing your different chakras. Start out by lying flat on a yoga mat. Bend your knees and make sure that your legs aren't touching and the distance between them is the same as the width of your hip. Now, place your hands on your sides and exert your weight onto your feet. By making use of your hips, you should slowly lift yourself off the ground. While doing this you can support your weight by making use of your palms. Move your arms to lie under your hips and interlock your fingers. Continue breathing in a relaxed manner. Hold this position for a while and when you are ready to move out of this position, do so by moving your hands to your sides first. Then you can lower yourself onto the ground and stretch out your legs in front of you. Relax your body and continue breathing slowly.

Corpse Pose

This is the best pose to practice and it doesn't require any effort from you. All you need to do is keep breathing in a relaxed manner. If this isn't enough reason to practice this pose, well, you can practice this even when you are sleeping in the comfort of your own bed. Just lie down on your yoga mat, keep your back flat on the mat and your feet at hips width from each other. Your hands should be kept close to your body and your palms should be facing upwards. Keep your eyes shut and breathe in a gentle manner to relax yourself. Pay attention to the way your breath flows in your body. Make a conscious effort to follow the flow of your breath in your body moving from your head to the tip of your toes. Stay in this position for a couple of minutes. When you feel that you are falling asleep, try increasing the pace of your breathing.

Plow Pose

This is one of the toughest yoga poses that you will ever come across. You will need to read all steps that are mentioned below. Read it a couple of times to get a better understanding and you need to make sure that you should take the precautions that are mentioned as well. Start out by grabbing two or three blankets and fold them into a rectangle. Stack the blankets on top of each other. Lie down on the blankets but make sure that your head rests on the floor. Only your back and your shoulders should be resting on the blanket. Your arms need to be by your side on your floor and bend your feet. Your heels should be touching your buttocks and your feet should be planted flat on the floor and exhale deeply. Slowly raise your hips off the ground and make sure that your thighs are moving inwards, towards your torso. Now you should move your pelvis and your lower back away from the floor, while moving your knees towards your face. Now bend your elbows and move your hands towards your lower back while your palms are flat to your back. Also make sure that your upper arms are resting on the blanket. Continue moving your pelvis upwards while making sure that your torso is perpendicular to the ground. Slide your hands downwards and do not let your elbows spread too far off from your body. You can maintain your balance by leaving your hands. Inhale slowly and straighten up your knees. Your toes need to be pointed towards the ceiling and press your arms and shoulders into the blankets to support yourself. Slowly lift your upper spine away from the floor and ensure that your shoulder blades are being held firmly against your back. Your thighs need to be in line with your torso and your chin should be pressed into your sternum but make sure that they are lying perpendicular to the ground. This particular pose is referred to as the Supported Shoulder Stand or the Salamba Sarvangasana. You need to hold onto this pose for about 30 seconds and then you can move into the plow pose. For this, you should slowly move away from your hip and exhale. Bring your legs backward over your head and lower your toes slowly so that they touch the ground. Also, make sure that your legs are fully extended. While keeping your toes planted on the floor, you should lift the top of your thighs and your tailbone as well upwards and towards the ceiling so that your torso is vertical to your hips. While doing this, you need to keep your chin drawn into your sternum. Now you can release your hands from your back and stretch out your arms. Make sure that your arms are right opposite your legs and use your hands to support yourself. Remove your hands only when you are sure that you will not fall out of the position you are in. Stay this way for a couple of seconds and then when you want to move out of this pose, you can move into the corpse pose you read about earlier.

There are some precautions that you should take while performing this exercise. You should not make any jerky movements because this could have an adverse effect on your spine. Also ensure that your movements are slow and gradual. Let the movements build gradually and you should avoid this pose if you are menstruating or happen to have any neck injuries.

Surya Namaskar

This is a really important exercise and this is one of the best exercises that you can practice for crown chakra. But you will have to work on your pranayama before you can start practicing this asana. You should stand on your yoga mat and place your feet together. You should balance your bodyweight equally on both your feet and expand your chest. Exhale and relax your shoulders. When you are breathing in, you should bring your arms closer to your chest and then fold them into a prayer position. Take a really deep breath in and lift your arms above your head. Make sure that your biceps rest next to your ears. Stretch onto the tips of your toes and you will need to make an effort to feel that pull throughout your body while you are stretching. Now push your pelvis forward and try to reach towards your back. Stretch and then bend your spine. Keep breathing out and bend forward. You should exhale completely and then make sure that your palms are touching the floor and your knees aren't bent. Take a deep breath in and then push your right leg as back as you can. Place your right knee on the floor and look up, straight ahead of you. Your left foot needs to be right in between your palms and breathe in slowly. Now move your left leg back into place. Your entire body needs to be in a straight line and your arms should be perpendicular to the floor. While exhaling you need to bring your knees to the floor. Now take your hips back slowly and when you are doing this slide a little forward and rest your chest along with your chin on the floor. Raise your buttocks and your hips a little off the ground. After this, raise your chest and move into the Cobra pose. For this, you will have to keep your hands firmly planted on the ground and raise your chest off the floor, imitating the way a snake would stand before it's ready to strike.

Your elbows need to bend and your shoulders should be away from your ears. Breathe out very slowly and lift your hips and your tailbone upwards. Now move your right knee in between your palm and stretch your left leg towards your back. Exhale slowly and bring your left foot forward. Then you can slowly start moving into your initial pose with your arms raised above your head and stretch yourself out. Finally, you can lower your arms to your side and relax a little.

Mountain Pose

This exercise is really easy; all you need to do is follow the procedure that is given here. Start by standing on your yoga mat with your feet together. Now you need to relax your shoulders a little and keep your arms resting by your side. If you feel that you are not able to balance yourself properly, then you can always keep your feet slightly apart. Now bend your knees slightly and then you can straighten them out. This will help you loosen your joints a little. The last step is to shift all your focus to a spot in front of you and just continue to focus on it.

The yoga poses that are mentioned above will definitely help you rectify any imbalances in your chakras and also help you open them. You just need to practice a little until you get a hang of it.

Chapter 8: The Hindu and the Buddhist tantras

The word 'tantra' references the traditions of both Hinduism and Buddhism as they co-developed their notion of chakra and meditation most likely around the 1st millennium AD. Classical traditions that were developed in India during this time described a 'subtle body' context, which connotes that we, as humans, live within the parallel dimension of psyche-mind reality that is invisible to us but very real. What vanishes when a person dies is this invisible energy that is synchronous with the breath, mind, and the emotions.

Different traditions in the Hindu Tanta wavered between a different numbers of these psychic-energy locations on the human body. The seven-part system that most people follow today (and that will be explored in this book) stems from this original Hindu tradition. The methodology was developed through a specific tradition within Hinduism called Shaktism. It is an important concept within a particular kind of yoga and meditation that is less practiced and known within the popularity of the Western World. These yoga poses and meditation practices focus on the energies of the chakras and how they associate with one another.

The traditional Buddhist Tantra generally teaches only four chakras. These chakras are considered psycho-spiritual constituents, each possessing their own meaningful correlation to cosmic processes and bodily counterpart. These chakras play a large part in the practice of Tibetan Buddhism, which is said to have not even existed without the establishment of these chakras. The goal is to sometimes combine particular yoga movements or meditation practices into the healing and clearing of the chakras (terms you will learn more about later) in order to completely free the self of negative conditioning

Chapter 9: Keeping Balance: Breathing Practices to Keep Your Chakras Open

Breath is significantly important to the quality of your energy and your chakras. Breath is life and the force that engages the flow of energy through your chakra system. The final chapter of this book offers you a series of breathing exercise for each chakra, designed to help you keep balance as you practice living with your energy.

We strongly encourage you to commit to using these breathing techniques on a regular basis. You can do them in the morning before work, or at the end of the day to clear all of the energy from your daily life or work schedule. They can be used in place of your yoga or fitness routine and can be a good way for you to practice your energy clearing techniques on a regular basis.

Bring breath to your chakras and awaken your energy within!

Breathe for the Root Chakra

1. Sitting on the floor, stretch your legs straight in front of you. Be sure to keep your back straight.

2. Place your hands to your shoulders and push your elbows out to the side in line with your shoulders.

3. Breathe slowly in through your nose. Lift your arms overhead and pull your knees up to your chest so they are pointing upward toward the sky. Make sure your feet stay flat on the floor and keep your sacrum planted to the ground while you reach up.

4. Begin to release your breath and lower your legs down, back into a straight position. Keep your spine straight while you bring your hands back to their original position on your shoulders, elbows pointed to the sides.

5. Repeat this cycle several times. If you feel comfortable, you can gain momentum, but be sure to keep in your comfort zone.

6. Remember to practice seeing yourself rooted to the Earth as you practice this exercise.

7. Ending this exercise, pull your legs into a cross-legged position. Sense the energy of your root chakra and consider it for as long as you need.

Breathe for the Sacral Chakra

Sit on the floor and draw your knees into your chest. Place your hands on the front of your knees. Your knees do not have to be against your chest, just slightly out from you, feet flat on the floor.

Breathe in through your nose and pull your sacrum forward, tilting your pelvis to make a curve in your lower back. Use your hands against the front of your knees to support your back.

Open your chest upward to the sky as you are pulling yourself forward and arching your back.

Breathe out and reverse the action to push the curve back, drawing your navel toward your spine and reversing the curve of your spine.

Repeat this cycle several times.

Bring your legs into a cross-legged position and shut your eyes. Return to a normal breath cycle. Meditate on the energy stirred and awakened in your sacral chakra and relax here for as long as you need.

1. Breathe for the Solar Plexus Chakra
2. Position your body in the same position you did for the second chakra. Place your hands gently on the front of your knees keeping them pulled close to your chest with your back straight.

3. Arch your back and pull your abdomen forward pushing your navel forward. Keep your back supported by keeping a hold of your knees with your hands.

4. Roll your torso from over to the left side, continuing all the way around. Pull your navel back into your spine and continue rolling back around to the front with your navel pushed forward. The idea is to create a smooth, circle roll.

5. Repeat this circle roll around starting from the front to the left side, and then back to the right side. Repeat several times.

6. Repeat again going in the opposite direction, several times.

7. You can gradually pick up speed but only if it feels comfortable for your spine. Don't overdo it and keep it slow if you need to limit your spinal movement.

The importance of this exercise is that you maintain focus on your breathing. Try to breathe in for the belly forward position, and then breathe out as you reach the navel-back position. Breathe in from the front to left to side, and breathe out from the back to right side, breathe in front…and so on.

Breath for the Heart Chakra

1. Sit with legs crossed on the floor or sit in a chair. Place your hands on your shoulders and push your elbows out so they are pointed to the side.

2. Take a slow and deep breath in. Twist your body to the right and lengthen and straighten your spine as you twist. Keep your abdominal muscles engaged.

3. Slowly breath out and twist your body all the way over to the left. Remember to keep your back straight and long. Engage your abdominal muscles engaged and chest wide open. Try not to arch your back.

4. Keep the breaths in and out slow and deep.

5. Repeat steps 1-4 several times.

6. Bring your back to normal resting position. Drop your hands down to your knees and breathe normally, keeping your eyes closed

7. Consider the energy of your heart and reflect on the feelings, thoughts or emotions that come up for as long as you need.

Breathe for the Throat Chakra

1. Sit with your legs crossed on the floor, or in a chair keeping your spine long.

2. Lace your fingers together and clasp your hands together. Keep your elbows pointing down towards your navel and touching together at their points. Place your clasped hands under your chin.

3. Inhale long and deep and push your elbows out to the side. Keep your fingers under the chin and woven together.

4. Letting the breath out, lift your chin and push your elbows back together. Keep your fingers as they were under your chin. Open your mouth and tilt your head back. Stick your tongue out for an extra stretch.

5. Make an audible sound while you breathe out. Any sound will do. Let it come naturally to you

6. Repeat this cycle of breath and motion several times.

7. Bring your head back to a normal resting position and breathe normally. Rest your hands in your lap, or on your knees. Consider the energy pulled into your throat chakra and

listen to the energy of your throat chakra for as long as you need.

Breathe for the Brow Chakra

1. Sit on the floor with your legs crossed or upright in a chair with your eyes closed Focus attention to your breath.

2. While breathing, envision opening a curtain or drapes hanging in front of your third eye to let light in. Imagine the drapes from your living room or bedroom if it helps you find the image you need.

3. Breathe in through your nose and then reach your hands out in front of you. Stretch your fingers wide and then open your eyes as wide as you can.

4. Reach your arms to the side while you hold your breath. Imagine as you reach your arms to the side that you are throwing the curtains open in front of a window. See a light, image, or color as you "open the drapes".

5. Breathing out, bring your hands to your face and cover your eyes. Picture in your brow chakra the image, shape, color or light that you envisioned with your eyes opened.

6. Repeat this cycle several times.

7. Return your breath to a normal pace for you. Rest your hands on your lap. Keeping your eyes closed, focus on your visualization. Practice seeing with your eyes closed.

Breath for the Crown

1. Sit in a chair or on the ground with legs crossed. Keep your spine long and chest open. Place your hands on your knees. Begin to concentrate on your breathing.

2. Places your palms together with your fingers pointed toward your chin and placed in front of your heart chakra.

3. Draw in a long, deep breath and then reach your arms and fingers up toward the sky with your palms still pressed together.

4. Breath out and reach your hands out to your sides in line with your shoulders.

5. Place your hands back in the prayer position in front of your heart. Begin your next breath in and start the next cycle over.

6. Repeat this exercise several times.

7. To finish this breath exercise, place your hands back in your lap, or on your knees and breath normally. Keep your spine straight. Reflect for however long you need to be silent and still.

Balancing Your Chakras

Balancing or aligning your chakras helps you to achieve a coordinated flow of energy within your whole being, making you feel some sense of restoration and wellness in the body as well as in the spirit.

Balancing the chakras needs to start with the root chakra and moving up towards the crown chakra.

Why balancing of chakras is important

For the energy within the body and mind to flow freely and easily from one point to another, the seven main chakras should be balanced and aligned. This makes an individual to have optimum body performance and mental health.

Balancing prevents the chakras from being blocked. Remember, once chakras are blocked, the affected person experiences emotional and mental upheaval. Where there should be calm and serenity, there usually is chaos.

The blocked chakras are caused by many things, but mainly, after you go through a harrowing experience, suffer a great loss like the passing away of a person that you held dear to your heart, an accident, a life changing event like divorce etc., they do cause a blockage in many if not all of your chakras.

Some people tend to be high-spirited due to balanced chakras. When they are well aligned, you will be active and lively, thus improving your performance at work, in bed, in school and in all of your daily activities.

What are the consequences of imbalanced chakras?

For proper communication between one chakra and another, one needs to keep the chakras balanced regularly. Yes, balancing the chakras should be done frequently with the aim of making sure all the chakras are in position such that they are not too open or too close to one another.

If the chakras are too open, they can cause overwhelming conditions that can make a person feel over-energetic, more active mentally or even too generous. This may lead to a person being easy to talk to but also too easy to convince hence anyone can take advantage of the situation. Such people with overactive chakras are easily taken advantage of.

When the chakras are too closed you find that one chakra is overworked by the other chakra. One chakra can also be underworked by another, thus causing an imbalance in the flow of energy within the body. For instance, if the sacral chakra is underworked by the root chakra, you will find that some of the important functions like sexuality, creativity and emotions become inhibited.

A person whose chakras are too closed may exhibit the traits of being too hard to communicate to; you find that such a person has low self-esteem. This makes him or her shy away from the public.

Imagine someone tying your feet and expecting you to walk a certain distance. That is exactly what happens when for example your root chakra is blocked, you will feel too slow with your movement or completely stuck to even lift your feet.

Blocked chakras can also make the energy flow within the body and mind to be limited within the area where the chakras are free, and not to the whole body as required. This may cause serious complications that may not be easily healed.

Once in a while, you will feel lacking in confidence to achieve some basic tasks. Yes, it is normal but it may also just mean that your chakras are imbalanced especially the root chakra. This calls for immediate balancing of the same.

There are some people that you meet and they seem to be insecure, they act all strange and timid. They are also very sensitive to nearly anything and they are very had to connect with, let alone to trust. Now that is a person with imbalanced sacral chakra. This makes an individual have some sense of insecurity, feeling like he or she doesn't belong.

Techniques to balance each of the 7 chakras

Each of the individual seven chakras need to be balanced if at all the body has to achieve optimum equilibrium.

Yoga healing for the root chakra

Get yourself a yoga mat, meditate, do your bikram, hatha, integral and many more for this is a very useful method to heal and balance your root chakra.

Yoga is highly recommended since other than just doing the postures, you can basically see (visualize) better while meditating which is also a very effective method of achieving root chakra balance.

Dancing is also a good way of balancing your root chakra. The sway of the hips, the legs moving gently and the feel of the moment keep your root chakra active.

Taking a bath is a basic routine, we do it because we have to - you wake up jump in the shower and you are done with the routine. Well, balancing the root chakra will need you to take an extra bath that is in accordance with the ritual.

This involves dipping yourself in waters that have been mixed with essential oils and herbs, this makes you entirely relaxed thus perfectly aligning your root chakra.

Yoga healing for the sacral chakra

"What you think is what you become." This is a famous quote from Napoleon Hill, the best-selling author of Think and Grow Rich. Coincidentally, we can use this very quote as a technique to balance the sacral chakra. Keep off the negative vibes, let go of the unhealthy emotions that you have been carrying around and drop all of your fears and insecurities. Take some time to identify what your ideal outcome or experience will look and feel like. And then repeat that experience in your head over and over. That's a way to fill your mind up with your desirable experiences which will eventually manifest in the real world.

Just like the root chakra is represented by the red color, so is orange for the sacral chakra, visualize the orange color, feel it on your sacral chakra and focus on that particular point. This will greatly improve its alignment.

The type of foods you eat also helps a great deal on how your chakras are balanced, for instance the orange color is depicted as the sacral color thus the foods with orange are important. Think of anything that is orange in color, either outside or inside. A pawpaw, oranges, carrots and many others should do the job.

Healing for the solar plexus chakra

Since this one is related to the yellow color, balancing solar plexus will need you to feed on foods that are yellow (like bananas).

You can also try dressing up to look neat and sharp. This has always been known to be a good confidence booster and thus it helps balance your solar plexus chakra.

Yoga for the heart chakra

View the nature and the environment and embrace the feeling that you're playing in a vast green park. Observe the green grass, the green leaves, the green canopy in the distance and so on. This will help in healing the heart chakra.

Feed on green vegetables and herbs. Anyway, the nutrients will do you a lot of good by removing toxins from the blood stream.

Aerate your home, let there be free flow of air. Forgive, forget, and by doing so you will feel some wellness start flowing in you, activating the heart chakra.

Yoga for the throat chakra

Anytime anything gets stuck in your throat, the first remedy is usually water, balancing the throat chakra needs you to take enough water too.

Other technique is to visualize the color blue since this is the color associated with the throat chakra. Also try to come to terms with your emotions, listen to yourself and get what you need for this chakra is hugely about communication.

Have a neck and shoulder massage once in a while for this will help relax your throat chakra.

Yoga for the Third eye chakra

A balanced third eye chakra can be helpful in developing your psychic abilities. To balance it, you need to consume foods rich in omega-3 fatty acids.

Have enough sleep and take adequate rest. This will help you to focus as well.

Take a moment and envision the whole week activities - what you did, what you encountered etc.

You can even have some daydreams. This will greatly help balance your sixth chakra.

Yoga for the crown chakra

This one is related to the violet color. So, visualize the color violet, try to feel it at the crown chakra spot. Close your eyes and imagine this color spreading from the crown of your head all the way down, to remaining parts of your body.

Go silent for a few minutes - this brings calm and removes stress. You can even try meditating. If you prefer guided meditation, check out the mobile app called "Headspace".

Use chakra stones and the most recommended is the clear quartz.

Do yoga, especially the ones that deal with breathing, close your eyes as though in a prayer but then let the inner voice guide you. That is how you get your crown chakra activated.

Various yoga poses and mudras

There are very many yoga positions and mudras including:

Lotus position

From a normal sitting position, put your feet on your thighs in an interlocking manner then make sure your torso is upright. Having done that, you will have assumed a lotus position otherwise known as the padmaasan.

This position helps in hip opening, flexibility of the knees and relay of knowledge throughout the body.

Corpse pose

Just like a corpse, lay on your back flat on the ground, stretch the whole body as far as it can go, legs few inches apart while arms few inches from the body.

It may seem easy but then this is the most difficult yoga position and it is usually done during the conclusion of a yoga class.

It is aimed at releasing stress and calming the body after concluding a yoga procession.

Lotus seal

This is not a position but a mudra where you put your hands together as though praying and then open them just the way that a flower blooms, while keeping the base of both hands in contact.

This usually helps to purify the soul

Handstand position

Just as the name suggests, it involves standing with one's hands, with your palms supporting your body upright against the ground. This pose can be a little bit scary but with regular practice, it is achievable.

It is very effective however for stabilizing your muscles.

Consciousness seal

While gently placing your arms on your thigh, fold out your arms, make an "O" sign with index and thumb while the other 3 fingers facing upwards and bent to a certain degree. This helps one release the inner prana. It's also called the Chin Mudra and is one of the most famous pose/mudra in yoga.

Conclusion

Don't forget that this book is just the beginning. The next step is for you to continue your practice. You have moved the first steps in this new path. You will soon find out that the beginning isn't the easiest part. But don't lose hope, maintain a positive mindset and stay focused. These practices are transformative in nature, so much so that you will visibly see your world change. This new life may be tough to adapt to, but once you have found a suitable practice you can rely on, you will be on your way to honing your skills.

The best way to begin with chakra opening and clearing is to meditate, and then take note of the symptoms that you feel are the most pervasive in your life. Then start with that chakra, moving to the next ones. Chakra balancing is a lifetime act. This means that your chakras do not get balanced and then stay balanced forever. You are a person who is active in the world; therefore, your emotions, physical body, spirit, and mood are going to be affected by it. Your chakras will always be in need of some balancing, depending upon the various occurrences in your life. This isn't something that is negative; it just simply is in the way we all have to keep up with physical exercises in order to maintain a good health condition. Eventually, you will have a specific routine, and you will figure out which activities of balancing benefit you the most.

No matter how many times a week you practice chakra work, whether it be meditation, yoga, finding chakra stones and crystals, or journaling, you are doing something positive for yourself. This is something that the universe will recognize. Keeping at it is something that will only benefit you, so should you feel discouraged, take stock of how you are feeling and move forward, deeper into the moment.

You have learned something new and are trying to integrate it into your life; this is going to take time. But since you have learned it, there is no way to get it out of your mind — a positive seed has been planted. You are going to notice the unbalancing of your chakras whether you like it or not. Even sitting reading this, you are probably vastly aware of the aches and pains in your body, your emotional issues, and troubles you have had for a long time that relates directly to certain chakras. If you raise your hands in the air right now and give them a stretch, your body will respond and so will your chakras!

The connection between the mind and body are undeniable, so doing chakra work on a daily basis is merely a way that you can begin learning more about yourself and allowing yourself to become one with what is around you and what is in you. So, fear not, good reader, you are moving forward along your path, and there is only positivity from here on out.

www.ingramcontent.com/pod-product-compliance
Lightning Source LLC
Chambersburg PA
CBHW050240120526
44590CB00016B/2171